Proceedings and Collections
Anti-cancer, anti-cancer metastasis research

THE NARRATE OF INNOVATION THEORIES

and

METHODS OF CANCER
TREATMENT VOLUME 2

Reform • Innovation • Development

The promising prospects of Immunomodulating drugs

Authors: Bin Wu, Lily Xu
Editors: Bin Wu, Lily Xu,
Translators: Bin Wu, Lily Xu

authorHOUSE

AuthorHouse™
1663 Liberty Drive
Bloomington, IN 47403
www.authorhouse.com
Phone: 833-262-8899

Published by AuthorHouse 09/08/2021

ISBN: 978-1-6655-3695-0 (sc)
ISBN: 978-1-6655-3696-7 (e)

Library of Congress Control Number: 2021913205

The human body is a hero.
All healing of the human body is an innate self healing
and is an inherent biological process.
Our health is controlled by our hands.
We are the drivers for our health.

The doctors are at their best with modifying, regulating, controlling the circumstances, the conditions under which we live, such as what type of diet, how much rest we have, how mch food we take, how much sleep we have, how much exercise we have, how much worry not justified, how much anxiety not justified.

It is very important in our lifes to stay in the present time, the present is a gift.
This is the way we should think of and this is the way we should live.

The main purpose for us to be healthy, it is that where we have the state of functional excellence which allow us to get the best mentally and physically and spiritually for ourselves (our organisum or our bodies).

<u>The cancer cure should be through regulation and controlling rather than killing</u>

In this book, I summary the new things and our past work together in the detail, <u>especially emphazie the medications for cancer treatment.</u>

Life is precious and let us prevent from cancer and other diseases.

Let us learn the things through hard work and others wisdom.

THE IMPORTANT CONCEPT OF CANCER TREATMENT

The cancer cure should be through regulation and control rather than killing.

Healing should be through regulation and control rather than killing.

The last step in curing cancer is to mobilize the reappearance of the host's control, rather than destroy the last cancer cells.

Cancer prevention is the same important as cancer treatment.

In another word, keeping our bodied healthy immune function is essential for completely curing cancer.

For the aboving concepts, there are some experiments to support them as the followings in brief:

From the father of medicine Hippocrates, "Everyone has a physician inside him or her; we just have to help it in its work. The natural healing force within each one of us is the greatest force in getting well. The next questions:

How can we wake up widely our inside physician?

Now along the technological rapid development, our human being works very hard to search for the good ways to live longer and to keep diseases free such as fasting, medication, meditation etc.

From Chinese book **"Huang Di Nei Jing"**, it is also said, *"the disease is not the inherent part of human body, which can be gained and also can be removed. If it can not be removed, it is because the method is not found.*

This means, the health is our normal state. If any disease happens to us, we should or could find the correct way to remove it. Our inherent part is health.

From Shong Han Theory, it is said, "*__losing grain can cure the diseases__*".

With thousand years people work hard to search for the ways for curing the diseases.

Where is the way for cancer theory?
How can it make cancer free from us?
How can we remove the cancer fear from us?

During our experiments, we surprisely found that cancer can disappear by their own or even if the cancer cells are injected into the body, the cancer will not grow at all.

Here some example of our experiments which were done as the following in brief, the detail and more experiment will be explained in detail in this book chapters:

1. From experimental studies, the process of cancer cell metastasis in the lymphatic tract was observed:

A. After transplanting $1X\ 10^6$ cancer cells under the skin of the inner side of the mouse paw pads, the animals were sacrificed at different times for local lymph node histological observation.

One hour after the transplantation of tumor cells, a single cancer cell was found in the marginal sinus of the cochineal lymph node, but no mitotic phase was seen;

After 3 hours, there are 3-5 groups of tumor cells in the marginal sinus of the cochineal lymph node, and mitotic phases can be seen;

After 5 hours, there are piles of cancer cells in the marginal sinus of the rouge lymph node, and some tumor cells have entered the middle sinus.

Twenty-four hours later, metastases had formed in the rouge lymph nodes. Scattered cancer cells were found in the middle sinus.

After 3-5 days, the popliteal lymph nodes have been occupied by metastatic tumor cells, and tumor cells and metastatic lesions were found in the second and third lymph nodes near the iliac artery and renal hilum.

Generally, metastases can be found in multiple lymph nodes after 3 days. Some cancer cells (such as Ehrlich's ascites carcinoma) form metastases only 5 days, and the metastases of rouge fossa lymph nodes can undergo degeneration and necrosis, and lymph node immune cells proliferate.

However, after 10 days, no cancer cells were found in the lymph nodes, and they were eventually destroyed by the host cells and disappeared.

The above experimental results suggest:

5 days after Ehrlich ascites cancer cells form metastases, the rouge lymph nodes may **undergo degeneration and necrosis**.

It indicates that the lymph node itself is a peripheral immune organ, which should be monitored and swallowed by cancer cells.

After 10 days, no cancer cells were found in the lymph nodes, which were obviously eliminated by the host's immune cells.

It is suggested that the treatment of anti-cancer metastasis can use the anti-cancer system and anti-cancer factors to protect and activate the host to destroy the invading cancer cells. The immune defense in the body can remove the cancer cells completely.

B. *Carry out experimental research on tumors and create cancer-bearing animal models*

A sterile tumor specimen was removed from the clinical operating table, and it was transplanted into experimental animals after 0.5h of warm ischemia. It was done more than 100 times (400 animals) without success. There was no any single animal which grew cancer yet.

However, when the thymus was first removed and then the cancer cells were transplanted in some mice, the cancer cells grew in the mice, which means after the removal of the main immune organ Thymus, it can promote the cancer cell growth. And this experiment was successful in the 210 animals.

Some injections of cortisone can reduce the immunity of mice and it can also promote the cancer cell growth so that the cancer cells can be transplanted successfully to the mice.

5 days after the thymus is cut and the cancer cells were transplanted, the large soybean nodules can grow after 5-6 days, and they grew to a large tumor of the thumb in 10-21 days.

Transplanted cancer can survive for 3-4 weeks, but it cannot be passed down to generations.

1. *Through this study, it is found that removal of the thymus can create a cancer-bearing animal model, and injection of cortisone can also help create a cancer-bearing animal model.*

2. *Research conclusions prove that the occurrence and development of cancer are related to the host's body immunity, and have a very obvious relationship with immune organs and immune organ tissue functions.*

3. *The results of this study confirmed that the immune organ thymus (Thymus, Th) and immune function have an extremely definite relationship with the occurrence and development of cancer.*

If the host Thymus is removed, it may be made into a cancer-bearing animal model, and if it is not removed, it cannot be a cancer-bearing animal model.

Injecting immunosuppressive drugs to reduce host immunity function will help create cancer-bearing animal models. Without injections of immuno-lowering drugs, cancer-bearing animal models cannot be created.

This result shows that immune organs and immunity are negatively correlated with cancer cell growth (during the cancer transplantation experiment and cancer implanation experiment) into solid cancer.

With immunodeficiency or reduced immunity, cancer cells of transplantation can implant and grow tumors without being swallowed or destroyed or damaged by the host's immune cells.

C. **From the animal experiments, cancer cells S_{180} 1×10^6 were** injected into Kuanming mouse through the tail vein, which were eliminated by 99% after 24-36 hours, and only less than 0.1 of cancer cells can be survived and can be grown and form the metastasis.

Who destroyed these 99% cancer cells?

It suggested that some of cancer cells were destroyed by the uncomfortable environment or the crash force or obstracting in the circulation of blood, however the most of the cancer cells after entering into the blood circulation mainly be destroyed by the host immune defences system such as the immune cells.

Hence, it should protect the host immune sysmentand should activate the host immune system function during treating the cancer and should not strike the host immune system and should not decreasethe host immune defense function.

In this book, there are many ways which are provided to protect the host immune functions.

In brief, healing is a biological process and is innate. Our body is the hero. There is no such things as chemicals, drugs, food and other ingredient that will take place of the living process of life.

All healing is self healing. Healing is not something that somebody else does to you. Healing is something you do for yourself.

The miracle is the living process and is it-self but what the doctor can do is the doctor can make decision about lifestyle which can enhance the person life or destroy the person life.

The choice or general speaking is yours and you have to make these decisions.

This is a book of the summary and reflection of the part of the past work for the cancer theorepy.

The extremely important concepts of cancer prevention:

1. _**Cancer is a disease that can be prevented**_ because now sinscien already proved that more than 90% of cancer occurrence are related to the environmental factors such as air, water, food, soil, and the social environment, etc.

2. Cancer is a diseae that threatens the human life so that the human _**should prevent and treat cancer**_; meanwhile it should realize that cancer can be prevented and cured; also it is very important to realize _**that cancer prevention should be put on the same attention and the same level at the same time**_ in order to stop and to eliminate the cancer occurrence at its source and before cancer happens.

3. _**It should do three early things: the early discovery, the early diagnosis, the early treatment. Cancer can be cured**_.

TABLE OF CONTENTS

To all my readers xv

About the Author 1 xxi

About the Author 2 xxiii

Preface xxv

Acknowledgements.. xxix

Part III

Walk out of the new path to conquer cancer.. 1

The Experimental research and anti-cancer research of immune
    pharmacology of Chinese medication on the molecular level combined
    Chinese and Western medicine 1

Walked out the new way of XZ-C immune regulation and control and
    molecular level combination of Chinese and Western medicine to
    conquer cancer 1

Walked Taking out the new way of using traditional Chinese medication
    to control and regulate the immune system, regulate immune vitality,
    prevent thymus atrophy, promote thymic hyperplasia, protect bone
    marrow hematopoietic function, improve immune surveillance, and
    combine Chinese and Western medicine to conquer cancer at the
    molecular level 1

(Anticancer medication research) 1

(The scientific research achievements) 1

Part IV

Walked out the new way to conquer cancer.. 75

1. XZ-C immunomodulatory anti-cancer treatment has been formed................... 75

2. For more than 20 years or over the past 20 years, the new path to
   conquer cancer has been walked out... 75

(The scientific research achievements) 75

TO ALL MY READERS

First, I deeply appreciate you for taking your precious time to open this book about the wellness of human beings.

Why do cancer and metastasis happen?
How should we treat it?
Can it be reversed by our bodies?
Can cancer be reversed and, if so, how?

During our experiments, some of the cancer in the rats disappeared after the cancer cells already moved to lymph nodes on the day of 8. When we injected cancer cells into mice and the lymph nodes had necrosis, eventually, the cancer disappeared.

All of these proved that our bodies had the ability to eliminate the cancer cells during our repeated experiments.

How can we help our bodies activate or enhance these abilities to remove cancer cells?

How can our body's physician be woken up to remove all cancer cells?

Technology has been dramatically developed, and many mysteries in the past have been clearly explained by scientific evidence. Many chronic diseases such as heart disease, cancer, metabolic diseases, and diabetics can be prevented and cured.

Cancer prevention is as important as the cancer treatment (it must be emphasized that prevention and treatment need the same attention and the same lever at the same time).

This book mainly emphasizes the medications which we use for treating cancer patients, especially the immunotherapy medications (the drugs' mechanism, the experiments, and the clinical verifications, etc).

In this book, many basic and clinical experiments in the lab proved and provided that cancer treatment should be through controlling it and should regulate the recovery of the body's ability of controlling the cancer, not through killing the final cancer cell. These experiments proved many of the new and important theories, such as:

The leading or guiding ideas of the new cancer model are:

Regulation and signal transmission between cells in cancer patients are disrupted rather than lost; the carcinogenesis is considered to be a *continuum with the possibility of reversal.*

Or it is considered that carcinogenesis is a continuum with the **possibility of reversal.**

Our body is constantly changing all the time and today's you is different from tomorrow's you.

Let us gather our knowledge:

1. *When I reviewed Greek medicine, the words from the father of medicine, Hippocrates gave me great relevance about our health:*

"Everyone has a physician inside him or her; we just have to help it in its work. The natural healing force within each one of us is the greatest force in getting well.

Our food should be our medicine. Our medicine should be our food. But to eat when you are sick is to feed your sickness."

- Hippocrates

This means our body has infinite healing wisdom.

How can we wake up completely this inner physician or search out this inside physician to get complete recovery?

In this book, we have written down some of this wisdom in detail, with some of the experiments in medication (the evidence), methods for cancer treatment, etc., which it can benefit our human health.

In this book, there are many medications which were tested and verified, and they had excellent effects on cancer patients.

Of course, there are many other ways such as fasting, exercise, meditation, etc.

2. *Technology has rapidly developed.*

Many things which we once thought of as impossible have now been achieved.

The understanding of life, such as physiology, pathogenetic pathophysiology, genetics, etc. grows fast as new technology and science develops rapidly after the knowledge and findings of humans increase.

Many mysteries of the living body have been explained and verified or confirmed by facts, such as:

1). Some cardiovascular diseases can be reversed, and *nitric oxide*, especially the **endothelium cell** is important for the vascular system to function well (1).

   It was found that good circulation is the key for our health, such as cancer metastasis and for our immune system (. As Dr. William Osler said: we are as old as our arteries.

2). Hyperinsulinemia (insulin resistance) and high carbohydrates are related to many diseases, such as diabetes (diabetes can be reversed completely), to the fibroid and to prostate diseases (2, 3, 4)

3). Our body can recycle to keep healthy, which is good for aging and many other diseases. It also has proven the concepts for many disease treatments, for a variety of diseases, which comes from the Nobel Prize in Physiology or Medicine 2016, awarded to Yoshinori Ohsumi "for his discoveries of mechanisms for autophagy." The concept gave evidence for fasting therapy for many diseases, such as aging, diabetics, cancer, and others more.

4). Our endocrine system is extremely important and related to many cancers and other diseases, such as estrogen (it is clear to relate this with breast cancer and other cancers, but especially those found in women), testosterone (it is one of the factors which is related to prostate cancer growth), *insulin (which is related to many conditions of the body)*, etc.

The human being is evolving and is now a hormonally modified human being. It is very important to keep the hormone balance between catabolism and anabolism, mainly by insulin (from the pancreas) and other hormones.

Our daily habits change our hormone levels so that if we change our habits, we can control our hormone balance to control our health situation. We will become the drivers for our health.

In addition, Hippocrates, the father of Western **medicine**, believed **fasting** enabled the body to heal itself. (He believed in the infinite healing wisdom inside human beings).

Paracelsus, another great healer in the Western tradition, wrote 500 years ago that "**fasting** is the greatest remedy, the physician within."

In brief, lifestyle changes are extremely important for our health, our aging, and our mind. This discipline is extremely important to keep good health.

3. *In Chinese <<Huangdi neijing>>, there were:*

The disease is not the thing belonging to our bodies, which can come and can be removed. If the disease cannot be removed, it is because the correct methods have not been found.

Persistence, persistence, and persistence!

During the time of COVID-19, I have stayed at home reviewing many medical textbooks about anatomy, biochemistry, immunology as well as clinical and experimental research data. One lecture I listened to repeatedly was given by a surgeon. One phrase that stuck out to me was, "Perhaps brains are important, but nothing and nothing is as important as persistence, persistence, and persistence.

"The road of science is not smooth, and similarly, neither is the road of life. After a long, challenging, and tearing road, this is finally here now."

How is this book new and what is it about?

This book focuses on cancer prevention and treatment, specifically on immune pharmacy.

We must accept the factors:

Technology is developing dramatically; the wonders of modern technology make many mysteries clear and clinical data has shown that many diseases can be cured and prevented by lifestyle changes and by our inside systems.

However, cancer is still a dangerous disease that threatens many people's wellbeing.

How can we help control these diseases?

What is the road that can cure and prevent these diseases?

This book will discuss a new way of controlling and preventing cancer. I hope you enjoy reading.

References:

(1). Prevent and Reverse Heart Disease: The Revolutionary, Scientifically Proven, Nutrition-Based Cure, by Caldwell B. Esselstyn Jr. Publisher : Avery; 1st edition (January 31, 2008)

(2). Hyperinsulinemia: An Early Indicator of Metabolic Dysfunction, Dylan D Thomas, Barbara E Corkey, Nawfal W Istfan, Caroline M Apovian.
Journal of the Endocrine Society, Volume 3, Issue 9, September 2019, Pages 1727–1747, https://doi.org/10.1210/js.2019-00065

(3). Diet-Induced Hyperinsulinemia as a Key Factor in the Etiology of Both Benign Prostatic Hyperplasia and Essential Hypertension?
Wolfgang Kopp, Mariatrosterstrasse 41, 8043 Graz, Austria.
Nutr Metab Insights. 2018; 11: 1178638818773072. Published online 2018 May 8. doi: 10.1177/1178638818773072 PMCID: PMC6238249 PMID: 30455570

(4). Uterine Leiomyomata in Relation to Insulin-Like Growth Factor-I, Insulin, and Diabetes.
Donna Day Baird,1 Greg Travlos,2 Ralph Wilson,2 David B Dunson,3 Michael C Hill,4 Aimee A D'Aloisio,1 Stephanie J London,1 and Joel M Schectman5
Published in final edited form as: Epidemiology. 2009 Jul; 20(4): 604–610. PMC2856640 PMID: 19305350

(5). International narcotics control board for 2009. New York: United Nations, 2010). Canadian Gazette. Controlled Drugs and Substances Ac

(6). The book<< new concept and new ways of treatment of cancer metastasis>>. Xu Ze, etc. Pressed in 2016 by authorhouse Inc. U.SA
Regulations Amending the Precursor Control Regulations (SOR/2005-365). 2005; 139(25). Available at: http://canadagazette.gc.ca/archives/p2/2005/2005-12-14/html/sor-dors365-eng.html (accessed 5 Apr 201 Canadian Gazette. Controlled Drugs and Substances Act: Regulations Amending the Precursor Control Regulations (SOR/2005-365). 2005; 139(25). Available at: http:// canadagazette.gc.ca/archives/p2/2005/2005-12-14/html/ sor-dors365-eng. html (accessed 5 Apr 201

(7). International Narcotics Control Board. Report of theInternational Narcotics Control Board for 2009. New York: United Nations, 2010. Canadian Gazette. Controlled Drugs and Substances Act: Regulations Amending the Precursor Control Regulations (SOR/2005-365). 2005; 139(25). Available at: http:// canadagazette.gc.ca/archives/p2/2005/2005-12-14/html/ sor-dors365-eng.html (accessed 5 Apr 201

Bin Wu, Lily Xu
04-27-21, in Timonium, Maryland USA

ABOUT THE AUTHOR 1

**A brief introduction to the first author
and the main translator and the editor**

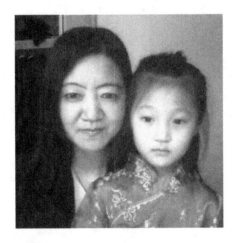

Bin Wu, MD, Ph.D., graduated from College of Yunyang of Tongji University of Medical Sciences for her MD degree; Studied her Master degree and her Ph. D degree in Sun Yat-Sen University of Medical Sciences. After she received her Ph.D., she worked as a Post-do4ctoral fellow in the Johns Hopkins Medical School and University of Maryland Medical School. She passed all of her USMLE tests and is going to do her residency training in America. She dedicated herself to oncology clinical and research. Her goal is to conquer cancer, which she believes this great contribution to our health. She has a daughter, named Lily Xu who gives great help with writing and editing and drawing all of the pictures in the books.

ABOUT THE AUTHOR 2

**A Brief introduction to the second author and
the editor and my only trustful advisor**

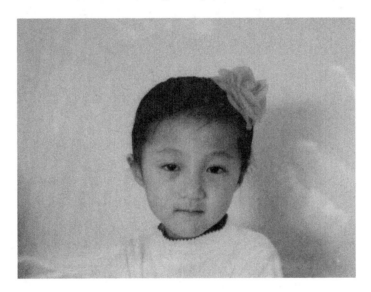

Lily Xu was born on November 17th 2006 and is in Advanced Biology Class in the high school since 2020. In 2020, she won the Robot designing model in Maryland and Math Model in Baltimore County in Maryland and she is in the Baltimore country honor banding. She helps with this book edition and others. She had an art presented in the Walter Art Museum in Baltimore at the age of 6; she got the fourth place trophy in the ES Double Digits or 24 and 24 games in the Baltimore County in Maryland; she got the first trophy in the BCPS STEM FAIR PHYSICS in Baltimore County; when she was in the sixth grade, she passed the advanced Math for 7th grade(which means the 8th grade math) test and moved the 8th grade math class and now she takes high school Math class; she loves the reading and the writing and she finished many seires of books and in 2019 summary she start to do volunteer job in the publish libarary. She got $9000 scholarship award for the Peabody music program in the Johns Hopkins University. She edits all of my books for the publishing and drew all of the pictures in this book. In 2018 and 2019 she was chosen into Baltimore county Middle school Honor Band. In 2018 the robotic team which she attended for years got designing-award from the Baltimore county so that this robotic team came to Maryland State for the Robotic contest in 2019. On January 19th, 2019 she got the Robotic designing award in Maryland. She edits all of my books for the publishing and drew all of the pictures in the book. In 2019 she was chosen by Baltimore County for one duel and one ensemble to play Clarion. Now she is in the nineth grade for her high school and while she was chosen to attend of Maryland state debate team in March 2021. She loves study and challenge and has execellent judgement. In 2021, she already won four medals for the different contests.

PREFACE

This monographs is not only written with a pen, *__but also made with real and hard work or done with actually working or performing.__*

The contents of these monographs all come from clinical practice experience and lessons, review, reflection, and **practice produces the reality and practice leads to know the truth**.

The contents of these monographs are all derived from the experimental research results of their own laboratories, and **the experiments produced results or achievement.**

The content of these monographs is a true record of scientific thinking and scientific practice from experiment to clinical, and then from clinical to experimental. The summary of experimental research and clinical verification data has risen to the essence of theory; meanwhile the new discoveries, new understandings, and new theories have been proposed. **All of these innovative theories of clinical practicability can be used to guide clinical treatment**.

All should be converted to clinical applications through translational medicine to guide clinical treatment and benefit patients.

The contents of these monographs:

They are all their own more than half a century of therapeutic practice experience and 30 years of experimental research materials. They are summarized, organized, and compiled into this book. The scientific research results and scientific and technological innovation series **are all their own materials, and some of them are international firsts. All of them are the original innovation. Some are internationally advanced and independent innovations, all with independent intellectual property rights.**

The content of this series of monographs:

Fully or completely is in line with or corresponds to the content of translational medicine.

Our 28-year scientific research route has been from clinical to experimental, clinical and experimental, and returns to the clinical to solve clinical practical problems. Our research model is completely in line with or matches this new medical research model.

Translational or transformation Medicine

Transformation Medicine recently develops rapidly and vigorously internationally.

This new medical research model advocates patient-centered, discovering and asking questions from clinical work, conducting in-depth basic research, and then quickly turning basic research results into clinical applications to improve the overall level of medical care and ultimately benefit patients.

Academician Chen Zhu, the former minister of the Ministry of Health, has analyzed the connotation of translational medicine:

First, translational medicine is a science that passes **through a two-way channel from laboratory to clinic and from clinical to laboratory for In-depth understanding the mechanisms of the occurrence and development of diseases and mechanisms of health protection promotion, and exploring new prevention and control strategies.**

Second, we **must transform scientific research results into clinical, public health, practical, interventional methods, technologies, and programs for their popularization.**

The World Health Organization proposes that medicine in the 21st century should not continue to use disease as the main research field, but should take human health as the main research direction.

Academician Chen Zhu pointed out:

The health service model should be transformed. It is necessary to shift from treatment-oriented in the late stage of serious diseases to prevention-oriented,

and move the gate forward and sink the center of gravity. Strengthening research in preventive medicine is a major issue in my country and the transformation of the global medical model.

The focus of my country's translational or transformation medicine research, the modernization and internationalization of Chinese medicine and Chinese medication is one of the key contents of my country's translational medicine research.

ACKNOWLEDGEMENTS

When I was close to finish this book, I recalled my parents dramatically because I realized their words and behaviour and spirit are so useful for me to live well. I looked at my parents and my childhood pictures and many beautiful momery showed up. I learned things from my parents. Now I realize that my father was such an excellent person on the healthy skills and the wisest doctor in my mind. He realized that the lifestyle of an individual is such an important thing for preventing and curing a disease. I learn to have a strong will.

If they were still alive, I would understand more medicine and do more things for others because I would get more things from their experience.

I thank my parents to enlighten me about the medicine since I started to understand things. My parents want me to do more contribution our societies.

When I was at the very young age, my father told me **how the bone morrow is important**. At that time, I didn't understand anything about immune system. My mother always told me something such **as garlic, ginger** function and why we eat them while I watched her cooked the dishes.

I thank my parents for trying very hard to lead me like to become a medical professional because both of them really loved what they dedicate and they wanted me to follow their footsteps. Both them let me come to the operation room to shadow them even far before I went to medical school. My father was excellent on many medical things. I miss my parents.

In addition, **I thank for Lily Xu who helps me editing all of my work and always give me the great and crystal idea and suggestion. She told me that the grammar should be paid attention to.** Thank for she studied hard by her own so that I can concentrate on this book.

Second, this book is for all of people who concern human being health.

We are deep grateful to all of people who like our new ways to improve our human being health. I appreciate to anyone who encourages me to continue working on my career. I thank for any good word which is encouraging me.

My daughter Lily Xu gives me many smart and creative ideas while we were finishing this book. **The characteristics of she loves the challenge** and her judgment always encourages me to continue working hard to move on. I learn the new things from her daily. I have to admit she is really smart on thinking things.

I would like to express our sincere gratitude to the following:

1. All of Authorhouse staffs

2. Dr. Xu Ze and other workers who were involved in cancer patient care.

3. Mrs. Bo Wu's family and Mrs. Tao Wu's famly

4. I deeply thank my only daughter Lily Xu, for her help with me and for her wisdom, for <u>her understanding me</u> and <u>for her update knowledge and for her loving learning</u>.

Bin Wu, M.D., Ph.D
04-29-2021 in Timonium, Maryland in USA

This book is the summary and collections of the part of the past work.

1. **The important concept *of cancer treatment*:**

   <u>The cancer cure should be through regulation and control rather than killing.</u>

   Healing should be through regulation and control rather than killing.

   The last step in curing cancer is to mobilize the reappearance of the host's control, rather than destroy the last cancer cells.

   <u>In another word, keeping our bodied healthy immune function is essential for completely curing cancer</u>.

2. **The important concept *of cancer prevention*:**

   Cancer prevention is the same importance as cancer treatment. It should put on the same attention and the same level at the same time. It is very important to do three early things: the early discovery, the early diagnosis, the early treatment so that cure can be cured.

   For the aboving concepts, we have some experients to support them in the following book content in the details.

Part III

Scientific and technological innovation
Scientific research achievement

Walk out of the new path to conquer cancer

The Experimental research and anti-cancer research of immune pharmacology of Chinese medication on the molecular level combined Chinese and Western medicine

—*Walked out the new way of XZ-C immune regulation and control and molecular level combination of Chinese and Western medicine to conquer cancer*

—*Walked Taking out the new way of using traditional Chinese medication to control and regulate the immune system, regulate immune vitality, prevent thymus atrophy, promote thymic hyperplasia, protect bone marrow hematopoietic function, improve immune surveillance, and combine Chinese and Western medicine to conquer cancer at the molecular level*

TABLE OF CONTENTS

The theoretical system of XZ-C immune regulation and control for treatment of cancer has been formed, and a new way of conquering cancer has been laid out for more than 60 years, and it has been undergoing clinical application and observation verification

Preface 5

1. The New discoveries in anti-cancer and anti-cancer metastasis research.......... 7
2. The experimental observation about the effect of tumor on immune
    organ thymus 12
3. The shape and location of the thymus.. 18
4. The structure of the thymus 21
5. The body's immune function 27
6. Thymus immune regulation function... 29
7. Exocrine function of thymus... 32
8. The influence of chemical drugs on the immune function of the body............ 33
9. The name and function of thymus hormone 34
10. Immune regulation: immune booster or promotor 35
11. Research progress in anti-cancer immunopharmacology of
    polysaccharides of traditional Chinese medicine.............................. 37
12. Characteristics of immunopharmacology of traditional Chinese medicine...... 40
13. The findings from experimental tumor research:............................... 43
14. Study on the mechanism of XZ-C immune regulation and anti-cancer
    Chinese medicine 46
15. XZ-C4 anti-cancer traditional Chinese medicine induced cytokine research 54

16. The experiment and clinical efficacy of XZ-C immune regulation and control anti-cancer Chinese medicine 57

17. XZ-C immune regulation and control anti-cancer Chinese medicine is the achievement or the result of the modernization of traditional Chinese medicine 66

PREFACE

The experimental surgery is extremely important in the development of medicine. It is a key to open the restricted medical zone. The prevention and treatment methods of many diseases are applied to the clinic only after many animal experiment studies and stable results have been obtained to promote the development of medical undertakings.

In order to have the development of science and technological innovation, the laboratory is the key condition.

It is deeply understood about the importance of the laboratory. Dr. Xu Ze is the first batch of college students after liberation. He has not studied for further training or studied abroad, but he has achieved many international-level achievements. The key is that he has a good laboratory.

In the 1960s, he participated in the open heart surgery laboratory with cardiopulmonary bypass.

In the 1980s, he established a laboratory for liver cirrhosis and ascites.

In the 1990s, he established the Institute of Experimental Surgery, with a focus on combating cancer. The animal laboratory has better equipment. There are animal experiments on mice, rats, guinea pigs, rabbits, dogs, monkeys, etc. There is a good sterilized operating room that can perform various major operations on the chest and abdomen and post-operative observation rooms for animals so that it was able to use various designs and ideas to achieve results or conclusions through experimental operations.

Therefore, the laboratory is a key condition, and the key is to build a well-equipped laboratory.

The university teachers should have dual tasks, one is to do a good job of teaching; the other is to develop science.

The university teachers should have good laboratories for scientific research, follow the scientific development concept, base on known sciences, explore unknown sciences, face future sciences, emerging disciplines, marginal subjects, interdisciplinary subjects, face the frontiers of science, strive for innovation and advancement, add bricks and tiles to the palace of science.

In summary, the experimental research and basic research are very important. Without breakthroughs in experimental research and basic research, it is difficult to improve clinical efficacy, and it is difficult to come up with new understandings, new concepts, and new theoretical insights.

The experiment is the key. *He has a good laboratory. He was the director of the Institute of Experimental Surgery. At the same time, he was also the director of clinical surgery.*

Therefore, the experimental research, basic research and clinical verification are convenient for overall planning.

Basic research in medicine is very important to make progress in the beat against disease. The experimental oncology is the basic science of cancer prevention and treatment research, which promotes the continuous and in-depth development of cancer research in my country.

The Institute of Experimental Surgery has conducted a series of experimental studies to explore the mechanism of cancer incidence, invasion, recurrence and metastasis. We have been in the laboratory for 4 years of experimental tumor research work. It was discovered from experimental tumor research:

1. *Thymus atrophy and low immune function may be the cause and pathogenesis of tumors.*
2. *How to prevent thymus atrophy?*
3. *How to regulate and control weakened immune function?*
4. *How to promote immunization?*
5. *How to "protect Thymus and increase immune function"?*
6. *Immune regulation should be carried out, combining Chinese and Western medicine at the molecular level, and the new path to combat cancer with Chinese characteristics should be walked out.*

The Experimental Study

1

The New discoveries in anti-cancer and anti-cancer metastasis research

The enlightenment of anti-cancer metastasis research

I am a clinical surgeon, why do I conduct research on cancer?

This is caused by the results of letters and visits to a group of postoperative cancer patients.

In 1985, I sent letters and visits to more than 3,000 postoperative patients with chest and abdomen cancer that I had done.

Results:

It was found that most patients had recurrence or metastasis within 2-3 years after surgery, and some even recurred or metastasized within a few months or one year after surgery.

From the results of the follow-up, **it is found that postoperative recurrence and metastasis are the key to the long-term effect of surgery.**

Therefore, an important question has been raised to us: that is, the *clinicians must pay attention to and study the prevention and treatment measures for postoperative recurrence and metastasis in order to improve the long-term postoperative efficacy.*

Therefore, it is necessary to conduct experimental research on the clinical basis of recurrence and metastasis. Without breakthroughs in basic research, it is difficult to improve clinical efficacy.

So we established an experimental surgery laboratory (Later in 1991, the Institute of Experimental Surgery of Hubei University of Traditional Chinese Medicine was established, with the research direction of conquering cancer).

We conducted research from the following two aspects:

One is animal experimental research; the other is clinical research.

On the basis of successful animal experiments, it is applied to the clinic for clinical verification.

After 28 years of hard work, a series of experimental research and clinical verification work have been carried out, and a series of scientific and technological innovation achievements have been made.

The new discovery

(1) The discovery from the follow-up results:

① *Postoperative recurrence and metastasis are the key to the long-term effect of surgery.*

② *Clinicians must pay attention to and study the prevention and treatment measures for postoperative recurrence and metastasis.*

(2) The discovery from experimental tumor research:

① The removal of the thymus (TH) can create a cancer-bearing animal model, and injection of immunosuppressants can also help the establishment of a cancer-bearing animal model.

The conclusion of the study clearly proves:

1. *The occurrence and development of cancer have an obvious positive relationship with the host's immune organ TH and immune organ tissue function.*

2. *It is difficult to make animal models without removing TH.*

3. *The experiment repeated many times and it is confirmed the experimental results.*

② Whether the immune system is low first and then the cancer is easy to get, or the cancer first and then the immune system is low:

The result of our experiment is:

1. Firstly, the immune system is weakened, and then the cancer is prone to occur and develop.

2. If there is no weakened immune function, it is not easy to be successfully vaccinated.

The results of this study suggest that improving and maintaining good immune function and protecting the good immune organ thymus is one of the important measures to prevent cancer occurence.

③ The animal models of liver metastasis established in our laboratory to study the relationship between cancer metastasis and immunity are divided into two groups A and B.

Group A uses immunosuppressive agents, but group B does not use the immunosuppressive agents.

The result was that the number of liver metastases in group A was significantly more than that in group B.

The results of this experiment suggest that metastasis is related to immune function, and the weakened immune function or the application of immunosuppressive agents may promote tumor metastasis.

④ When our laboratory conducted experiments to explore the impact of tumors on the immune organs of the body, it was found that as the cancer progressed, the thymus glands gradually atrophy.

After the host's thymus gland was inoculated with cancer cells, it showed acute progressive atrophy, cell proliferation was blocked, and its size was significantly reduced.

The results of this experiment suggest that tumors can inhibit the thymus and cause immune organs to shrink.

⑤ Through experiments, we also found that if some experimental mice were not vaccinated, or the tumors grew very small, the thymus glands did not shrink significantly.

In order to understand the relationship between tumors and thymus atrophy, we experimented with transplanting solid tumors in a group of experimental mice when they grew to the size of their thumbs, the cancer was removed or cut off. 1 month later, the thymus will not further shrink. In other words, an autopsy revealed no further atrophy of the thymus gland after 1 month.

__Therefore, we speculate that solid tumors may produce an unknown factor to inhibit the thymus, which requires further experimental research.__

⑥ *__The above experimental results prove that the progression of the tumor causes the thymus to shrink progressively. So, can we take some measures to prevent the host thymus from shrinking?__*

__Therefore, we further design and want to use the immune organ cell transplantation to restore the function of the immune organ.__

In our laboratory, to explore how to stop the atrophy of the immune organ thymus during the prevention of tumor progression, to find ways to restore the function of the thymus, and to rebuild the immune function, **the experimental study of adoptive immune reconstruction of fetal liver, fetal spleen and thymocytes in mice was carried out.**

The results showed that the combined transplantation of S, D, and L cells has a complete tumor regression rate of 40% in the short term and 46.67% in the long-term. Those who have completely resolved the tumor will have long-term survival.

⑦ When we were investigating the effects of tumors on the spleen, the immune organs of the body, we found that the spleen had an inhibitory effect on tumor growth in the early stage of the tumor, and the spleen also showed progressive atrophy in the late stage of the tumor.

The results of this study suggest that the effect of the spleen on tumor growth is bidirectional, with a certain inhibitory effect in the early stage and loss of the inhibitory effect in the late stage.

Spleen cell transplantation can enhance tumor suppression.

This is a new discovery in experimental research and a very important discovery that should be further studied.

In summary, from the above series of experimental studies, it is found that thymus atrophy and low immune function may be one of the causes and pathogenesis of cancer.

It should go further in-depth research about

a. *the function and tissue structure of the thymus;*

b. *the decrease of immune function;*

c. *how to promote immunity;*

d. *rebuild the immune system,*

e. *and how to protect the Thymus and promote immunity.*

Let's review the structure and function of the thymus, and look for new ways and methods for cancer treatment.

The Experimental Research

2

The experimental observation about the effect of tumor on immune organ thymus

It is generally believed that the immune function status of the body affects the occurrence, development and prognosis of tumors, and at the same time, **tumors will also inhibit the immune status of the body. The two are mutually cause and effect, and are complicated.**

When the author was conducting animal experiments on the effect of spleen on tumor growth, many changes were observed about the immune organs such as thymus and spleen in the tumor-bearing mice.

It seems that there is a certain regularity during these or a certain pattern in the meantime.

In order to further explore the relationship between tumor and spleen and thymus and its regularity, the following experiment was designed to dynamically observe the changes in the thymus, spleen and transformation rate of lymphocytes in tumor-bearing mice at different periods to explore the regularity during the period.

【Materials and Methods】

(1) The experimental animals and grouping

Forty Kunming mice were randomly divided into 4 groups, aged 40-50 days and weighing 15-18g. No distinction between male and female.

Group I: healthy control group, healthy mice without cancer cells. Thymus, spleen and peripheral blood were taken for experimental observation after execution.

12

Group II: 0.1×10⁷ Ehrlich ascites tumor cells were inoculated into the abdominal cavity and sacrificed after 3 days for observation.

Group III: inoculated with tumor cells (same as above), sacrificed on the 7th day for observation.

Group IV: On the 14th day after tumor cell inoculation, the patients were sacrificed for observation.

Take the autopsy results of 100 tumor-bearing mice after the spontaneous terminal death in the Chapter 22 experiment (the experimental study of the effect of the spleen on tumor growth) as the result of the changes in the thymus and spleen of advanced tumors.

The average diameter of the thymus in late-stage tumor-bearing mice is (1.2 ± 0.3) mm, and the average weight is (20 ± 5) mg, and the texture is hard.

The spleen is extremely atrophic, with an average weight of (60 ± 12) mg, hard texture, grayish-white color, significantly reduced growth centers, and fibrosis.

(2) The experimental method

The mice in each group were put to death by eyeballs and bleeding at the planned time. Each mouse was left with 1ml of whole blood (anticoagulated with heparin) for performing a lymphocyte transformation test, and then immediately dissect the mouse to observe the tumor infiltration area, ascites volume and the involvement of various organs, and focus on the naked eye to observe the anatomical morphology of the thymus, spleen, and lymph nodes, completely remove the thymus and spleen, and measure their volume with a vernier caliper. Then weigh them with an analytical balance and send them for medical examination.

【Experiment Results】

(1) The weight of the mouse thymus at different stages after inoculation with tumor cells

See Table 1

Do analysis of variance on Table 1, see Table 2. The results of Table 1 and Table 2 are represented by curves, and the thymus weight change curve is drawn (Figure 1). The weight of the thymus on the 25th and 30th days in the figure is from the results of the experimental part in Chapter 22.

Table 1
The comparison of thymus weight of experimental mice in each group (mg)

Group	Group I normal group	3 days after group II inoculation	Group III 7 days after vaccination	The 14th day after group IV inoculation
Xij	72.8 50.0 56.4 96.4 77.4 100.7 87.5 76.8 112.7 51.0	78.2 83.4 89 68 74.8 95.4 11.50 56.4 43.0	90 66.0 85.4 106.5 51.7 77.8 73 60 49.4	40.0 32.2 39.8 23.5 38.0 36.0 46.0 20.0 55 20
ΣX	781.07	703.2	736.3	350.5
Ni	10	9	10	10
X	78.17	78.13	73.63	35.05
X	66261.79	58566.66	57033.75	18467.25

Table 2
Performs analysis of variance on table 1

Source of variation	SS	V	MS	F	P
Between groups	12967.10	3	4322.36	12.85	<0.01
Within groups	11777.12	35	336.48		
Total	24744.22	38			

It can be seen from Table 1, Table 2 and Figure 1 that the thymus of the tumor-bearing mice showed regular changes. Within 7 days after inoculation, the thymus had no obvious changes in naked eyes, but the weight had begun to decrease.

After days, it showed acute progressive atrophy.

In the late stage, the diameter of each lobe of the thymus was reduced from the normal 5-8mm to about 1mm, and the weight was reduced from 76.1mg to 20mg. The texture became hard, and the function was also reduced or even lost.

It shows that the body's cellular immune function is increasingly manipulated and inhibited as the tumor progresses, causing the immune function to become weak, and the tumor grows faster and faster.

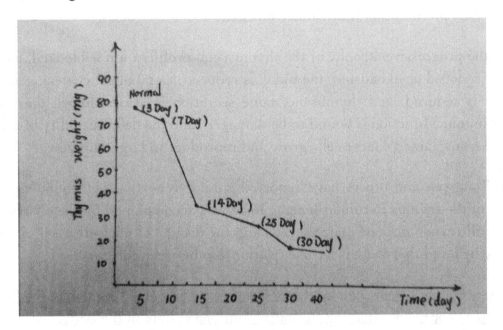

Figure 1
Thymus weight change curve

(2) Pathological changes of thymus

Thymus presents progressive atrophy throughout the course of the disease.

On the 3rd day after inoculation with tumor cells, the thymus is slightly smaller and slightly paler in color.

On the 7th day after inoculation, the thymus is significantly atrophied, cell proliferation is blocked, and mature cells are reduced.

And to the late stage of the tumor, the thymus gland is extremely atrophy, the size is about the size of a sesame seed, the diameter is 1mm, and the texture becomes hard.

(3) About the effect of tumor on thymus

The experimental results showed that after inoculation with tumor cells, the thymus was immediately suppressed and progressively atrophied throughout the course, so the thymus immediately lost its anti-tumor immune effect. It was observed in the experiment that the thymus undergoes morphological and structural changes soon after the tumor cells are inoculated, and the whole course of the disease shows progressive atrophy. In the late stage of the tumor, the weight of the thymus decreased from 78.13±13.2mg to 20±5mg, and the volume decreased from 5-8mm in diameter to 1mm. Cell proliferation is obviously blocked.

Due to the progressive atrophy of the thymus, cell proliferation is blocked, mature cells are reduced or exhausted, the index is reduced, metabolism is weakened, cell viability is reduced, and thymus hormone secretion is also reduced, the body's cellular immune function is bound to be damaged, and the defense ability of mice is low. The transplanted cancer cells grow and reproduce in large numbers.

Zhang Tongwen and others have reported similar reports. They found that the atrophy of the thymus in tumor-bearing mice was accompanied by the obstruction of the proliferation of bone marrow cells and the decline of nucleated cell viability, and they believed that there is a close relationship between the two.

It can be seen that tumors can inhibit or damage the immune function of the host in many aspects or ways, affecting the entire immune system of the body.

This group of lymphocyte transformation rate experiments showed that after inoculation with cancer cells, the lymphocyte transformation rate decreased progressively, and decreased by more than 50% in the late stage, which also indicated that the cellular immune effect was suppressed.

As for how the thymus of tumor-bearing mice is suppressed and shrinks, further experimental research and observation are needed.

The thymus also produces a variety of thymic hormones to promote the differentiation and maturation of immune lymphoid stem cells.

Although the thymus is a lymphatic organ, due to the existence of the blood thymus barrier, the thymus does not come into direct contact with antigenic substances and exert its effect.

Therefore, it is not stimulated by tumor-specific antigens to grow and enlarge. The tumor produces and secretes immunosuppressive factors, but it can act on the thymus, causing it to shrink and function.

In the immunotherapy of malignant tumors, many doctors are devoted to the development of this field with great interest.

Since the 1980s, due to the rapid development of immunology and biotechnology, it has provided opportunities for immunotherapy for cancer patients. The biological response adjustment theory has been proposed and the fourth treatment program except surgery, radiotherapy and chemotherapy has been established. It is the biological therapy of tumor (BRM).

The use of biomodulators to treat tumors may hopefully promote the development of new immunotherapies that are effective for tumors.

In short, the host and tumor are a pair of contradictions, which always exist in the entire process of tumor occurrence and development.

When the body's immune system is functionally healthy, the body's cellular and humoral immune response to tumors can limit and eliminate tumors. On the other hand, the growing tumor has a lot of influence on the body's immune system, inhibits the body's immune function, and promotes the development of tumors.

3

The shape and location of the thymus

The thymus is cone-shaped and can be divided into two asymmetrical left and right lobes.

The thymus is soft in texture and has a long flat strip shape. The two lobes are connected by connective tissue (Figure as the following).

The size of the thymus varies greatly between age groups.

In the late embryonic development and newborns, the thymus grows rapidly.

From birth to 2 years old, it is the best period for thymus development. The weight is 5-20g.

With age, the thymus continues to grow and grow, but it grows more slowly than in the postnatal period, reaching 25-40g in puberty.

After puberty, the thymus begins to shrink and degenerate.

Adult thymus still maintains its original shape, but its structure changes greatly, lymphocytes are greatly reduced, and thymus tissue is mostly replaced by adipose tissue.

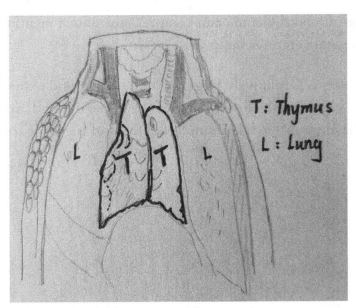

Figure   The morphological position of the thymus in children

The adult thymus is located behind the sternal stem on the front of the mediastinum. The rear side is adjacent to the innominate vein and the aortic arch, and both sides are adjacent to the mediastinal pleura and lungs.

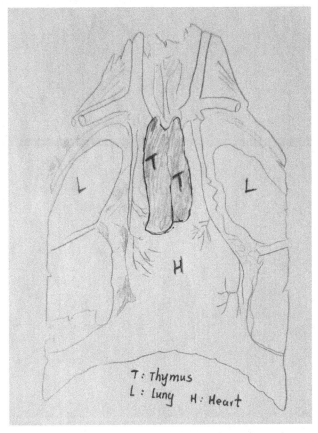

Figure   Upper mediastinal organs and pericardium, thymus

Thymus enlargement and thymoma can compress the above-mentioned organs, and corresponding clinical symptoms appear.

In children, the thymus is relatively large, with the upper end extending to the base of the neck, some reaching the lower edge of the thyroid gland, and the lower end extending into the anterior mediastinum to the front of the pericardium.

4

The structure of the thymus

(1) Envelope:

The surface of the thymus is covered with a connective tissue envelope, which is composed of dense collagen fiber bundles, elastic fibers and matrix, etc. The connective tissue fiber bundles in the capsule extend into the thymus parenchyma, dividing the thymus into many lobules. The lobule is surrounded by the cortex and the deep side is the medulla. There is a scaffold composed of reticulocytes between the two (as the following Figure).

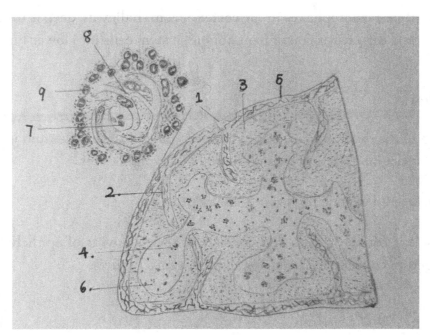

Figure   The structure of the thymus in children

1. *Thymus lobules;*
2. *Lobular interval;*
3. *Upper cortexon the thymus;*
4. *Thymus corpuscles;*
5. *Film or cover of thymus;*
6. *Medulla;*
7. *Keratinized epithelial cells and debris;*
8. *Epithelial cells;*
9. *Thymocytes*

(2) Cortex:

The cortex of the thymus is located around the lobules and is composed of dense lymphocytes and epithelial reticular cells.

The lymphocytes in the superficial layer of the skin are larger and belong to primitive lymphocytes.

The lymphocytes in the middle layer are medium in size, and the inner layer is mostly small Lymba cells.

There are scattered macrophages in the cortex. From shallow to deep is the process of proliferation and differentiation of hematopoietic stem cells into lower lymphocytes.

(3) Medulla:

The medulla of the thymus is located in the deep part of the lobules and is composed of epithelial reticular cells and a small number of lymphocytes.

There are scattered thymic bodies in the medulla.

The corpuscle is round or oval, and consists of several layers of epithelial reticular cells arranged in concentric circles (as the following Figure).

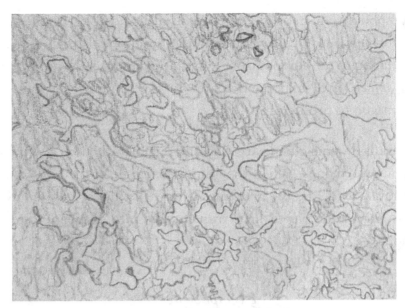

Figure   Thymus Medulla

The picture shows scattered thymic corpuscles distributed in the medulla

Thymus function

The function of the thymus is more complicated. The thymus is a lymphatic organ and has the function of an endocrine gland. Some authors include it in the endocrine system. Its main function is to cultivate and produce T lymphocytes and secrete thymus hormones. The cultivation of T cells in the thymus requires a suitable internal environment.

The epithelial reticulum unitary cell of the thymus can secrete a variety of hormones:

Thymosin (thymosin), thymopoietin (thymopoietin), thymosin (thymulin), thymic humoral factor (THF), ubiquitin, etc.

These hormones and ***macrophages and interlaced cells*** in the thymus, etc. form a microenvironment for cultivating T cells, of which thymosin and thymosin can be:

1. *To promote the differentiation of lymphoid stem cells into T cells,*
2. *Stimulate T cell proliferation,*
3. *Stimulate the hypothalamus to secrete ACTH and LH;*
4. *Thymopoietin can induce T cell differentiation;*
5. *Other hormones have a synergistic effect on the early division of T cells and the promotion of T cell maturation.*

Primordial lymphoid stem cells have no immunity, and after further development, they are transformed into T cells with immune functions. It then migrates through the blood circulation to the surrounding lymphatic organs, such as **_lymphatic tissues, lymph nodes, spleen_**, etc., and participates in the immune response after being activated by antigen to proliferate.

Although the adult thymus glands atrophy and degenerate, they still have the ability to secrete thymus hormones. When the lymphatic tissue of the body is destroyed, T cells are greatly reduced, and the lymphatic stem cells that circulate into the thymus with the blood circulation can still be transformed into T cells under the action of thymus hormone.

T lymphocytes

T cells derive their name from this organ Thymus where they develop (or mature).

What is a T cell?

A **T cell** is a type of lymphocyte. T cells are one of the important white blood cells of the immune system, and play a central role in the adaptive immune response.

T cells can be easily distinguished from other lymphocytes by the presence of a T-cell receptor (TCR) on their cell surface.

T cells are borne from hematopoietic stem cells, which are found in the bone marrow and the developing T cells migrate to the thymus gland to mature.

Differentiation and development of lymphocytes in thymus

After migration to the thymus, the precursor cells mature into several distinct types of T cells, whose differentiation also continues after they have left the thymus.

The groups of specific, differentiated T cell subtypes have a variety of important functions in controlling and shaping the immune response.

Phenotypic changes during T cell differentiation and development

Immune-mediated cell death is one of these functions, and it is carried out by two major subtypes:

CD8+ "killer" and CD4+ "helper" T cells, which are named for the presence of the cell surface proteins CD8 or CD4.

CD8+ T cells, also known as "killer T cells", are cytotoxic, which means that they are able to directly kill virus-infected cells, as well as cancer cells.

CD8+ T cells are also able to use small signaling proteins, known as cytokines, to recruit other types of cells when mounting an immune response.

A different population of T cells, the CD4+ T cells, function as "helper cells".

These CD4+ helper T cells function is to indirectly kill cells identified as foreign:

which determine if and how other parts of the immune system respond to a specific, perceived threat.

These CD4+ also use cytokine signaling to influence regulatory B directly, and other cell populations indirectly.

Regulatory T cells are yet another distinct population of T cells that provide the critical mechanism of tolerance, whereby immune cells are able to distinguish invading cells from "self". This prevents immune cells from inappropriately reacting against ones' own cells, known as an "autoimmune" response.

For this reason, these regulatory T cells have also been called "suppressor" T cells, which can also be co-opted by cancer cells to prevent the recognition of, and an immune response against, tumor cells.

It is currently known that the main factors that induce T cells to differentiate and mature in the thymus include:

1. *Thymus stromal cells (thymus stromal cell, TSC) directly interact with thymocytes through adhesion molecules on the cell surface;*

2. *Thymic stromal cells secrete a variety of cytokines (such as IL-1, IL-6, IL-7) and thymic hormones to induce thymocyte differentiation;*

3. *The secretion of multiple cytokines (such as IL-2, IL-4) by thymocytes also plays an important role in the differentiation and maturation of thymocytes.*

In addition, epithelial cells, macrophages and dendritic cells in the thymus play a decisive role in the self-tolerance of thymocytes during differentiation, MHC restriction and the formation of T cell functional subsets.

5

The body's immune function

In particular, the functions of cellular immunity and T lymphocytes gradually decline with age, and the thymus gradually undergoes structural and functional degeneration after adulthood.

__The thymus is the central organ of immune function and the base for T lymphocyte differentiation and maturation__.

Thymic epithelial cells produce and release thymosin (thymosin), which plays an important role in the differentiation of precursor T lymphocytes into mature immunocompetent T cells.

__Thymus is also the earliest organ in the body to degenerate__.

It begins to shrink after sexual maturity, and its ability to produce and secrete thymosin gradually declines with age.

The study of the thymus began in the early 1960s, when it was found to be closely related to immune function.

Miller et al. (1960) found that the immune function of dethymic animals (newborn mice) was underdeveloped and the number of circulating T cells was significantly reduced.

For 50 years, the thymus has been recognized as the central organ of the immune system of the animal body.

It is the earliest organ that matures the body. The structure and function of the thymus reaches a peak when it reaches sexual maturity, and then gradually shrinks and degenerates with age.

The immune function is gradually replaced by the **spleen and other lymphatic system tissues i**n adult animals.

The thymus is the core tissue for the development of T lymphocytes, and at the same time it is the base for the production of various immune factors (lymphokines, cytokines).

Thymosin is the main immune regulator secreted by it. There are many kinds of thymosin (peptides). The products are used for clinical and experimental research.

There is a special journal abroad called "thymus", which regularly publishes reports on thymus research and clinical treatment.

6

Thymus immune regulation function

From the beginning, it was considered to be a single self-regulating system independent of other physiological systems, and it has been developed to date that it has been considered that the thymus and neuroendocrine system are interconnected, unified and coordinated functional network systems.

In the late 1970s, Besedovsky (1977) proposed the neuroendocrine immune network theory (NIM), which has been recognized as the core idea that guides the thymus and immune function. The thymus forms a three-point and one-line connection with the central nervous system and the peripheral immune response system.

The central cerebral cortex, hypothalamus, and pituitary gland are the superior regulatory centers;

Peripheral lymphoid organs and tissues, lymphocytes and cytokines are the regulators and executive units of the lower-level immune network;

__the intermediate hub station is the thymus, which can be called the middle line of NIM.__

__The NIM pathway can be divided into three:__

(1) Downline, that is, from the center to the middle line and downline units.

(2) Upline, each cytokine feedback information to the central part from the downline; or *__On the up line, each cytokine from the down line feeds back information to the central part;__*

③ The midline pathway, with the thymus as the main axis, accompanied by the spleen and other lymphoid tissues and bone marrow progenitor cells, or ***the midline pathway, with the thymus as the main axis, is accompanied by the spleen and other lymphoid tissues and bone marrow progenitor cells.***

Recent studies have proved that the thymus plays an important role in NIM activities.

For example,

Fabres (1983) put forward the concept of "thymus-neuroendocrine network" as the figure:

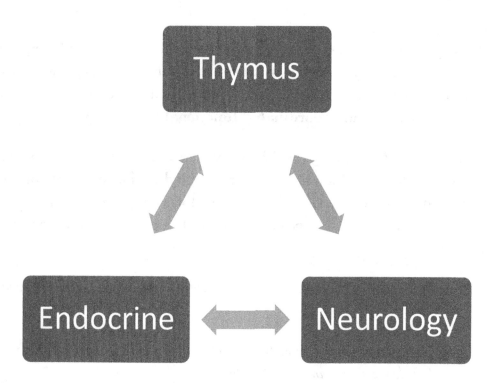

Goldstein AL (1983) put forward the idea of "neuroendocrine-thymus axis", which can be said to express the special significance of thymus in NIM network.

The thymus begins to degenerate after sexual maturity, and the secretion of thymosin and other hormones also decreases, which hinders the differentiation of T lymphocytes and reduces the body's immune function.

The main cause of aging in humans and mammals is closely related to the atrophy and degeneration of the thymus. With age, the thymus gland naturally shrinks and life gradually ages. The thymus gland is an important factor affecting the body's immune level.

Experiments have proved that the removal of the thymus in adult rats (2 months old) can accelerate the decline of their own immune function and aging. The immune activity of splenic lymphocytes in rats (2 months old) decreased significantly after 6 months of thymic removal, which was only 51.6% of the same age without thymus.

7

Exocrine function of thymus

Thymus hormone activity can be detected by biological identification methods. The experiments have shown that the vitality of thymus hormone decreases with age, and decreases with thymus atrophy.

It cannot be detected in the serum of animals with the thymus removed. The thymus is the main source of thymus hormone.

Thymus hormone is a hormone secreted by thymocytes and has the effect of regulating immune function.

Thymus is an important tissue of the body's immune function, secreting and producing thymosin (hormones such as thymulin), and secreting IL-1 and IL-2 and other interleukin components to regulate the internal function and cell viability of the thymus.

At the same time, it is regulated by the prolactin secreted by the pituitary gland.

It can be seen that the current research on immune regulation of the thymus has provided preliminary evidence, showing that exogenous endocrine hormones (such as prolactin, growth hormone, thyroxine, etc.) can induce the rejuvenation of the decayed thymus and maintain immune regulation.

Thymus recession can be reversed, which is the common research and development prospect of modern immunology and endocrinology.

8

The influence of chemical drugs on the immune function of the body

Cyclophosphamide (Cy) or hydrocortisone (HC) is a commonly used drug in clinical practice, which can cause a decline in immune function. Long-term injection can cause atrophy of the thymus, spleen and lymph nodes, and significantly decrease immune function.

In short, although Cy and HC have a certain inhibitory effect on immune function, such as Cy is used for 3 weeks(W), the thymus has atrophy; after 6W, the spleen also began to shrink; at 6-12W, the proliferation of peripheral blood T lymphocytes decreased significantly.

9

The name and function of thymus hormone

Since the famous scientists Good and Miller first reported that the function of the thymus is the "central" organ of the body's immune system in the early 1960s, cellular immunology has developed rapidly.

The hypothesis that the thymus secretes hormones was put forward in the early 1970s.

Several "presumptive" but not yet confirmed thymus hormones or hormone-like components have come out one after another. They are all peptide components extracted from the whole thymus.

Recent studies have shown that thymic epidermal cells (TEC) are cells that produce thymic hormone components, which can be divided into two categories:

Interleukins (ILs) and thymosin peptides.

Foreign studies have proved that there are 4 kinds of thymus hormones:

(1) thymosin- a;
(2) thymulin;
(3) thymopoietin;
(4) thymichumoral factor (THF)

Thymulin is a 9-peptide binding component that requires zinc binding to have biological activity.

Thymus components are mostly extracted from bovine thymus in foreign countries.

10

Immune regulation: immune booster or promotor

As far as the current situation is concerned, immune boosters can be divided into several categories due to different sources:

1. The first type of immune enhancer is firstly derived from microorganisms. For example:

Fungal glucan:

The ingredients containing ß-1, 3-glucoside chain have been shown to have good clinical effects. They can promote Mφ to kill bacteria and tumor cells and induce the release of monokine, such as interleukin 1 (IL-1), Tumor necrosis factor (TNF), colony stimulating factor (CSF), etc.

2. The second major type of immune booster is thymus extract.

The peptide ingredients are extracted from animal thymus, which there are many products produced and showed up in each country (including my country). All of which have immunopharmacological activity, also called ***thymus hormone.***

Zinc thymulin complex is an active ingredient secreted by thymic epithelial cells. A variety of other crude thymus extracts have clinical effects. Its main function is to enhance the vitality of T cells in the body, but it has no effect on generating new T cells..

In other words, activating T cells can enhance the body's anti-microbial, anti-tumor vigor and delay the decline of the immune function of aging animals.

Clinically, it is mostly used to treat chronic infectious diseases and tumors.

3. **The third major category of immune-promoting agents is the recombination of cytokines that were developed in the 1980s.**

These biologically active factors have achieved significant benefits in clinical treatment, the most prominent of which are: IFN-r, IFN- a, IL-2 (IL-1 to IL-2), TNF, rCSF (such as GM-C SF).

This can be said to be a major innovation or breakthrough in immunopharmacology. Recently, monoclonal antibodies (Mabs) and human gene antibodies (H-Ab) have appeared. These new components can be classified as recombinant peptide immune substances.

Significant progress has been made in the purification of the above-mentioned multiple immune-promoting substances, and a variety of effective products are now available, among which there are not too many chemical substances that have proved to have clinical therapeutic effects.

The following parts are the research on Immunopharmacology of Traditional Chinese Medicine:

11

Research progress in anti-cancer immunopharmacology of polysaccharides of traditional Chinese medicine

<u>Anti-tumor research on Lycium barbarum polysaccharide, Polyporus umbellatus polysaccharide, Poria cocos polysaccharide, Lentinan, Yunzhi and Ganoderma lucidum polysaccharide, Tremella polysaccharide.</u>

<u>Mechanism and prospect of anti-tumor effect of polysaccharide drugs</u>

1. **Research progress in anti-cancer immunity of traditional Chinese medicine polysaccharides:**

Polysaccharides can improve the body's immune surveillance system, including natural killer cells (NK), macrophages (Mφ), killer T cells (CTL), T cells, LAK cells, tumor infiltrating lymphocytes (TIL)), interleukin (IL) and other cytokines to achieve the purpose of killing tumor cells.

Although many polysaccharides have a certain anti-tumor effect when used alone, two immunopotentiators, including two polysaccharides, have a higher curative effect. The use of polysaccharides with chemotherapy or radiotherapy can further improve the curative effect.

2. **The research overview and progress**

Thomas and Burnet's immune surveillance theory proposed that the body's immune system has the function of eliminating tumor cells produced by cell mutations in order to maintain a single cell type of each cell.

The body's immune surveillance system for tumors includes cellular immunity and humoral immunity, and cellular immunity is particularly important for tumor rejection.

Immune cells that perform cellular immune functions include natural killer cells (NK) and macrophages (Mφ). Recently, LAK cells and tumor infiltrating lymphocytes (TIL) have been proposed, the latter having 50-100 stronger anti-tumor effects than LAK cells Times, played a stronger role. If these effector cells are inhibited, it is difficult to play the role of the immune surveillance system.

Elston reported that there were only 3 deaths in 19 choriocarcinoma patients with cellular immune response, and 13 deaths in 24 patients with no immune response or significantly reduced immune response, indicating that the level of immune function of the body plays an important role in tumor treatment.

The prevention and treatment of tumors by enhancing the immune function of the body is undoubtedly a promising research field.

According to the research progress of polysaccharides at home and abroad and relevant information, polysaccharide drugs include LBP, on the one hand, it can play a role in anti-bacterial, anti-viral, anti-tumor, anti-aging, anti-radio-chemotherapy side effects and anti-autoimmune diseases; It may also have various physiological activities such as lowering blood pressure, lowering blood lipids, anti-vomiting, and lowering blood glucose.

These aspects will also be important directions for the in-depth research and application development of LBP.

Compared with other polysaccharides, LBP is composed of a glycopeptide with strong action, small dosage, good water solubility, stability and easy absorption by oral administration. It can be considered as a highly effective immune T cell adjuvant.

However, LBP is still a crude extract, and it needs to cooperate with phytochemical experts to purify and modify LBP, including degradation into oligosaccharides and oligosaccharides of different molecular weights, and sulfated polysaccharides. It is expected to further improve the immune activity of LBP, in order to find a newer immune activity drug.

Immunity is closely related to aging. Further studies by many scholars have found that the main reason for the deterioration of cellular immune function during aging is that the thymus gland shrinks with age.

Therefore, some people have proposed that the thymus gland is the biological clock that controls the immune function during aging.

LBP is exactly to act on the thymus, the main link of aging immunity. The main experimental proofs are as follows:

1. LBP mainly acts on thymic T cells;

2. Ding Yan and other reports pointed out that LBP can promote the increase in the number of mature T cells in the thymus, and enhance the "emptying" function, so that thymocytes can metastasize and proliferate to the periphery, play the regulatory role of the thymus immune center, and enhance the role of disease resistance and anti-aging;

3. Our experiments have proved that the elderly mice drink LBP aqueous solution daily. After half a year, the thymus glands of the control group atrophy, and the thymus glands of the LBP group recover and the weight increases, but they have not reached the normal adult level.

This fact suggests that LBP can reverse aging thymic degeneration.

Based on the above, we can clearly understand the relationship between the thymus and aging.

12

Characteristics of immunopharmacology of traditional Chinese medicine

Compared with immunopharmacology of western medicine, immunopharmacology of traditional Chinese medicine has its own characteristics or advantages, but also has its own shortcomings. The advantages of Chinese medicine immunology are roughly as follows:

The first is that long-term clinical managers have accumulated a large number of prescriptions that have the effect of regulating the body's immune function, especially tonic Chinese medicines generally have the benefit of regulating immune vitality.

There are abundant sources of traditional Chinese medicines. In recent years, studies have increasingly proved that traditional Chinese medicines are effective medication in the long-term clinical treatments. After extraction, they can have obvious pharmacological effects (including immunomodulatory effects). The research process saves people, saves time and has high benefits.

Secondly, Chinese medicine contains multiple active ingredients, whether single medicine or prescription, unlike western medicine (synthetic medicine) which is a single structure substance.

The role of traditional Chinese medicine is multifaceted. In addition to regulating the immune function, it also has certain effects on the overall functional systems and organs. And these functions are interrelated and combined.

The role of traditional Chinese medicine in regulating immune function is generally tonic, that is, within the normal regulation range, with two-way regulation as the main feature.

Tonic drugs can be called immunomodulatory drugs, which cause non-specific immune responses.

Tonic traditional Chinese medicines all have the effect of regulating the immune function of the body.

Under general experimental conditions, there is a correlation between dose and benefit, especially in normal healthy animal experiments.

When the animal is at a low level of immune activity (such as dethymic animals, aging animals, or under the suppression of the chemotherapy drug cyclophosphamide, and tumor animals), tonic drugs improve the body's immunity more significantly.

Immunopharmacology is a marginal subject formed by the combination of immunology and pharmacology.

Immunopharmacology of Chinese medicine occupies a particularly important position in my country's immunopharmacology.

Immune pharmacology of Chinese medicine can be understood as a new subject that is grafted from traditional Chinese medicine and modern immunopharmacology.

As early as the 1970s, Professor Zhou Jinhuang had been calling for the establishment of pharmacology of integrated traditional Chinese and western medicine in my country, and clearly proposed to study and clarify the pharmacological effects of traditional Chinese medicine based on the theory of traditional Chinese medicine.

Traditional Chinese medicine theory has its obvious overall view, emphasizing the balance of the body and maintaining balance when the internal and external environment changes.

If balance and coordination are lost, the body will develop symptoms.

Modern medicine also places great emphasis on the stability of the internal environment.

The regulatory factors for the stability of the internal environment are the three major systems of nerves, endocrine, and immunity.

These are both self-contained systems and independently play their respective regulatory roles. At the same time, they are interconnected and interact with each other, so as to achieve the purpose of maintaining a relatively stable internal environment.

"Nerve, endocrine, immune, and regulatory network" (NIM network) is currently a research hotspot in immunopharmacology.

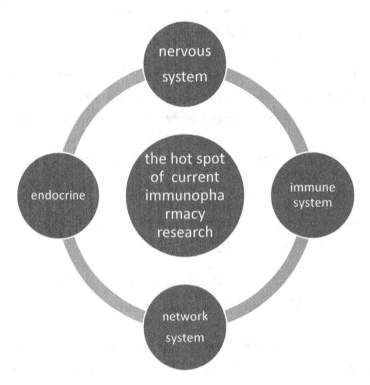

<u>Professor Zhou Jinhuang has developed NIM thinking through a lot of research work, and believes that the concept of "NIM" has broad practical significance, conforms to the laws of life science, and coincides with the overall thinking system of traditional Chinese medicine.</u>

Extensive and in-depth research on the effect of Chinese medicine on the NIM network can greatly develop the relevant basic theories of Chinese medicine and enable Chinese medicine to enter the world faster.

The molecular research on Chinese medicine is as the following:

13

The findings from experimental tumor research:

(1) Removal of the thymus (Thymus, TH) can create a Dutch animal model

(2) Tips of experimental results:

Metastasis is related to immunity, and low immune function may promote tumor metastasis;

(3) The experimental results found:

After being inoculated with cancer cells, the host's thymus showed acute and progressive atrophy, cell proliferation was blocked, and the size was significantly reduced;

(4) The experimental results found:

When the transplanted solid tumor in the experimental mouse grows to the size of the thumb, it is removed. One week later, an autopsy revealed that the thymus did not shrink;

(5) Our laboratory is exploring the atrophy of the immune organ thymus during the prevention of tumor progression, looking for methods of immune reconstruction, and adopting mice to carry out the experimental research of adoptive immune reconstruction of fetal liver, fetal thymus, and fetal spleen cell transplantation.

The results show:

The combined transplantation of S, T, and L cells showed a complete regression rate of 40% in the short-term and 46.67% in the long-term.

From the above experimental studies, it has been found that thymus atrophy and low immune function may be one of the pathogenesis and pathogenesis of tumors. We should start from the body's immune function, especially cellular immunity, T lymphocyte function, and thymus immune regulation function. It is to discuss or explore at the level and seek methods of immune regulation and control.

In view of the development of immunopharmacology of traditional Chinese medicine, the theory of traditional Chinese medicine has its obvious holistic view or the concept of the whole picture, emphasizing the balance of the body, maintaining balance when the internal and external environment changes, and losing balance, the body will have disease symptoms.

Modern medicine also places great emphasis on the stability of the internal environment and the regulation of the stability of the internal environment. The factors are the three major systems of nerves, endocrine and immune systems.

"Nerve, endocrine, and immune regulation network" (NIM network) is the current research hotspot in immunopharmacology.

There are a large number of traditional Chinese medicines that can regulate the immune function of the body, especially tonic Chinese medicines generally have the benefit of regulating immune vitality.

In the past 28 years, we have conducted a series of experimental studies,

a. *Looking for new anti-cancer, anti-cancer metastasis, preventing thymus atrophy, and increasing immunity from natural medicine,*

b. *Look for new anti-cancer drugs from natural medicines;*

c. *Looking for anti-metastasis and anti-relapse drugs;*

d. *Look for drugs that only inhibit cancer cells but not normal cells;*

e. *Look for Chinese medicine to prevent thymus atrophy,*

f. *Adjust the regulatory relationship between the host and the tumor,*

g. *Drugs to prevent recurrence and metastasis.*

The existing anti-cancer drugs suppress the immune function of the patient, suppress the hematopoietic function of the bone marrow, suppress the thymus, suppress the bone marrow, make it lose the immune monitoring, and make the cancer further develop.

Therefore, research must be strengthened to ensure that all anti-cancer drugs used must enhance immunity and protect immune organs, not drugs that suppress immunity.

14

Study on the mechanism of XZ-C immune regulation and anti-cancer Chinese medicine

__Looking for new anti-cancer and anti-metastasis drugs in natural medication (Chinese medicine)__

In the experimental work, our laboratory has carried out anti-tumor screening experiments in tumor-bearing animals on 200 kinds of traditional Chinese herbal medicines that are traditionally regarded as "anti-cancer Chinese medicine" in batches for a long time.

As a result, it was found that only 48 of them have certain or even better inhibitory effects on the proliferation of tumor cancer cells.

After optimized combination, then through in vivo tumor suppression experiments in tumor-bearing animal models such as **liver cancer, lung cancer, and stomach cancer, etc**, they were composed of XZ-C$_{1-10}$ particles, XZ-C$_1$ can significantly inhibit cancer cells, but does not affect normal cells, XZ-C$_4$ can protect the Thymus and increase immune function, promote immune function, XZ-C$_8$ can protect the bone marrow to produce blood.

XZ-C immune regulation and control of Traditional Chinese medicine can improve the quality of life of patients with advanced cancer, increase immune function, strengthen physical fitness, increase appetite, and prolong survival.

__With the deepening of research on traditional Chinese medicine, many traditional Chinese medications are known to have regulatory effects on the production and biological activities of cytokines and other immune molecules. This is of great__ *significance for elucidating the immunological mechanism of XZ-C immune regulation and anti-cancer Chinese medicine at the molecular level."*

(1) XZ-C anti-cancer Chinese medication can protect immune organs and increase the weight of thymus and spleen

The role of XZ-C Chinese medication in protecting immune organs is exerted by the following active ingredients in the medication:

1. XZ-C-T (ASD)

Use its extract (1g per milliliter equivalent to the original drug) 15g/kg, 30g/kg of ferulic acid suspension 12.5mg/kg, 25mg/kg to the mice every day for 7 days, **all of which can significantly increase weight of mouse thymus and spleen. Especially in the high-dose group, the effect is more obvious.**

Injecting its polysaccharide into the abdominal cavity of mice can also significantly reduce the atrophy of thymus and spleen caused by prednisolone.

2. XZ-C-O (PMT)

1. The extract PM-2 was administered to normal mice with PMT6g/ (kg·d) decoction for 7 days, **which can significantly increase the weight of the mouse thymus and abdominal lymph nodes**, and can antagonize the immune organs caused by prednisolone weight drops.

2. Giving 15-month-old mice its water decoction (concentration 0.5g/mI) 6g/kg for 14 days can significantly **increase the weight and volume of the mouse thymus, thicken the cortex, and increase the cell density.**

3. The combined use of PM and Astragalus can significantly promote the proliferation of non-lymphocytes and help improve the microenvironment of the thymus.

3. XZ-C-W (SCB)

SCB polysaccharides can **increase the weight of the thymus and spleen of normal mice**.

Gavaging with it can also increase the weight of the thymus and spleen in mice that are immunosuppressed by cyclophosphate.

4. XZ-C-M (LLA)

Infusion of LJA water decoction to mice for 7 days can significantly increase **the weight index of mice thymus and spleen.**

5. XZ-C-L

1. The thymus glands of 15-month-old mice degenerate significantly.

2. **Astragalus injection can increase the thymus glands**. Under light microscope, the cortex thickens and the cell density increases.

(2). The effect of XZ-C anti-cancer Chinese medication on the proliferation, differentiation and hematopoietic function of bone marrow cells

The following active ingredients of XZ-C Chinese medicine have an effect on bone marrow hematopoietic function.

1. XZ-C-Q (PMT)

The effect of extract (PM-2) and Z-C-Q (LBP) on the proliferation of normal mouse bone marrow hematopoietic stem cells (CFU-S):

The experimental mice were given PM-2 intravenously at a dose of 50 mg/(kg·d) X 3d or LBP at a dose of 10 mg/ (kg· d) X 3d. The test mice were killed alive on the 9th day. It was found that the administration group was small The number of CFU-S in the spleen of mice increased significantly. The CPU-S of PM-2 group and LBP group were 121% and 136% of the control group, respectively.

It can be seen from the above experiments that PM-2 and LBP have a significant promotion effect on the hematopoietic function of normal mice. Experiments have shown that:

In the recovery process of hematopoietic function damage caused by cyclophosphamide in mice, *__PM-2 and LBP first stimulate the proliferation of granule progenitor cells, then the bone marrow nucleated cells increase, and finally it promotes the recovery of peripheral granulocyte count.__*

2. XZ-C-D (TSPG)

Ginseng total saponins are the effective components of ginseng to promote hematopoietic function. It can promote the recovery of peripheral red blood cells, hemoglobin and femoral bone marrow cells in myelosuppressed mice, increase the division index of bone marrow cells, stimulate the proliferation of bone marrow hematopoietic cells in vitro, and make them enter the active proliferation Cell cycle (S+G2/M phase).

TSPG can promote the proliferation and differentiation of pluripotent hematopoietic stem cells (CFU-S) and myeloid hematopoietic progenitor cells.

TSPG can induce the production of hematopoietic growth factor (HGF).

3.XZ-C-H (RCL)

Rehmannia glutinosa can promote the recovery of red blood cells and hemoglobin in blood-deficient animals, accelerate the proliferation and differentiation of bone marrow hematopoietic stem cells (CFU-S), and have significant hematopoietic effects.

Continuous injection of Rehmannia glutinosa polysaccharides into mice's abdominal cavity for 6 days can significantly promote the proliferation and differentiation of hematopoietic stem cells and progenitor cells in the bone marrow of mice, and increase the number of peripheral blood white blood cells.

4. XZ-C-J (ASD)

Polysaccharides have no obvious effect on the red blood cells and hemoglobin of normal mice, but injection of ASD polysaccharides into radiation-damaged mice has obvious effects on the proliferation and differentiation of pluripotent hematopoietic stem cells (CFU-S) and hematopoietic progenitor cells of various lines. But the decoction has no obvious effect.

5. XZ-C-E (PEW)

Yunlingin (small molecule compound extracted from Yunling polysaccharide) can enhance the production of colony stimulating factor (CSF) and increase the level of peripheral blood white blood cells in mice, and can prevent the decrease of white blood cells caused by cyclophosphamide. The recovery speed is accelerated, and the effect is stronger than that of sodium ferulate.

6. XZ-C-Y (PAR)

Its polysaccharide can significantly resist the leukocyte-reducing effect of cyclophosphamide, increase the number of bone marrow cells, promote CSF-induced bone marrow cell proliferation, promote the recovery and reconstruction of hematopoietic function in X-ray irradiated mice, increase hematopoietic stem cells, increase the number of bone marrow cells, and increase leukocyte.

(3) XZ-C anti-cancer Chinese medicine can enhance the immune function of T cell

The effective ingredients and functions of XZ-C Chinese medicine are as follows:

1. XZ-C-L (LBP) can significantly increase the percentage of peripheral blood lymphocytes in mice. A small dose of LBP (54Omg/kg) can cause lymphocyte proliferation, indicating that LBP has a significant effect on T cell proliferation.

   With 50mg/(kg·d) X7d as the optimal dose, there is no obvious promotion effect below this dose, but the effect will decrease if the dose exceeds this dose.

   Oral LBP can increase the lymphocyte transformation rate of tumor patients with weak physique and low white blood cell.

2. XZ-C4 has the function of regulating the immune system, can activate the T cells in the collective lymph nodes, and stimulate the secretion of hematopoietic growth factors in the T cells.

   Among the crude drugs that make up XZ-C4, the hot water extract of rhizome of Atractylodes japonicus has obvious effect of stimulating lymph node cells, which is considered to be the basis of XZ-C4 immune regulation.

(4) Activation and enhancement of XZ-C anti-cancer Chinese medicine on NK cell activity

Natural killer cell (NX cell) is another type of killer cell in human and mouse lymphocytes. It can kill certain cells without antigen stimulation or antibody participation.

It has an important immune function, especially in the body's immune surveillance function.

NK cells are the first line of defense against tumors and have a relatively broad anti-tumor spectrum.

NK cells have a broad-spectrum anti-tumor effect, which can kill tumor cells of the same line, the same species and xenogenes, and are especially effective against lymphoma and leukemia cells.

NK cells are an important type of immunoregulatory cells, which have a regulatory effect on T cells, B cells, bone marrow stem cells, etc., and by releasing cytokines (such as IFN-a, IFN-y, IL-2, TNF, etc.) the body's immune function is regulated by NK cells.

The specific active ingredients in XZ-C Chinese medicine are as follows:

1.XZ-C-X

Fangfeng (SDS) can enhance the activity of NK cells in experimental mice.

When combined with IL-2, NK activity is higher. It shows that Fangfeng polysaccharide promotes the activation of NK cells by IL-2 and helps to improve the activity of NK cells.

LBP can enhance the T cell-mediated immune response and NK cell activity in normal mice and cyclophosphamide-treated mice.

Intraperitoneal injection of LBP can increase the proliferation of mouse spleen T lymphocytes and enhance the killing function of CTL. The rate of special killing increased from 33% to 67%.

2. XZ-C-G

Glycyrrhizin (GL) induces IFN in animal and human blood, and also enhances NK activity.

Clinical trials by Abe et al. showed that intravenous injection of 80 mg GL increased the activity of NX cells by 75% in 21 patients.

Injecting 0. 5mg//kg of GL can enhance the activity of NK cells in the liver.

3. ZCL (AMB) solution can significantly promote the activity of mouse NK cells in vivo and in vitro, and it can directly induce mouse IFN-y (AMB) to treat effector cells at a certain concentration ((0.1mg/mi)).

Cordyceps alcohol extraction can enhance the activity of mouse NK cells in vitro and in vivo.

0.5g/kg, 1g/kg, and 5g/kg can significantly enhance the activity of mouse NK cells.

(5) The effect of XZ-C anti-cancer Chinese medicine on interleukin-2 (IL-2)

XZ-C anti-cancer Chinese medicine specific active ingredients and functions:

1. XZ-C-T

EBM polysaccharides can significantly enhance the production of human IL-2 at 100ug/ml.

(EBM) At high concentrations (2500ug/ml/ and 5000ug/ml), it shows inhibition. Epidermis polysaccharides injected continuously subcutaneously for 7 days can significantly improve the ability of ConA-induced mouse thymus and spleen cells to produce IL-2.

2. XZ-C-Y

PEP polysaccharides have strong immune activity. It can promote the production of IL-2. For S180 tumor mice, the IL-2 production capacity of mouse spleen cells can be significantly improved.

3. XZ-C-D

Ginseng polysaccharide has a significant promoting effect on the induction of IL-2 by peripheral monocytes in healthy people and patients with kidney disease, and it is in a dose-effect dependent relationship.

(6) XZ-C anti-cancer traditional Chinese medicine induces and induces interferon(IFN)

IFN has a broad-spectrum anti-tumor effect and immunomodulatory effect. IFN can inhibit tumor cell proliferation, and IFN can activate NK cells and CTL to kill tumor cells. At the same time, IFN can also cooperate with TNF, IL-1, IL-2 to enhance the anti-tumor effect.

The effective ingredients and functions of XZ-C anti-cancer Chinese medicine:

① XZ-C-Z

CVQ polysaccharide 250mg/kg or 500mg/kg can significantly increase the level of IFN-Ý produced by mouse splenocytes.

② XZ-C-D

Ginsenosides (GS) and ginsenosides (PTGS) can induce human whole blood cells and monocytes to produce IFN-a and IFN-ýI, and can also restore normal IFN-ý and IL-2 in tumor-bearing mice.

The ASH polysaccharide stimulated the acute lymphocytic leukemia cell line S180 and the acute myeloid leukemia cell line S7811 to produce IFN titer that was 5-10 times higher than that of the normal control group.

③ XZ-C-E

Light methyl tuckahoe polysaccharide has a variety of physiological activities such as immune regulation, induction of IFN, indirect antiviral, and reduction of radiation side effects. The IFN induction kinetics experiment on S180 leukemia cell line with 50 mg/ml methyl tuckahoe polysaccharide showed that the potency of induced interferon induced by light methyl tuckahoe and other polysaccharides in each phase was significantly higher than that of conventional induction.

④ XZ-C-G (GL)

It can induce IFN activity. While it was to give Intraperitoneal injection of GL33Omg/kg to mice, IFN activity reached the peak after 20h.

15

XZ-C4 anti-cancer traditional Chinese medicine induced cytokine research

(1) <u>XZ-C4 anti-cancer Chinese medicine can induce endogenous cytokines</u>

① According to experimental research, XZ-C4 has a variety of immune enhancement effects and is closely related to the induction of endogenous cytokines.

② XZ-C4 can inhibit the reduction of white blood cells, granulocytes and thrombocytopenia.

③ XZ-C4 not only has a direct effect on the production of granulocyte macrophage colony stimulating factor (GM-CSF) through interleukin-1ß (IL-1ß). And it can enhance various cytokines such as tumor necrosis factor (TNF) and interferon (IFN). The latter may be an indirect mechanism.

④ In cancer patients, Th1 cytokine that regulates cellular immune function has decreased, while XZ-C4 can increase it. It is effective for anemia and leukopenia after chemotherapy.

⑤ Experimental analysis found that XZ-C4 not only protects the bone marrow, but also has a direct effect on the differentiation of cancer cells through cytokines.

<u>In short, XZ-C4 exhibits various cytokines due to autocrine (autocrIne), thereby inducing cancer cell differentiation and natural death. The so-called autocrine means that the substances secreted by oneself in turn act on oneself.</u>

<u>Looking to the future, XZ-C4 may become an induction therapy for cancer cell differentiation.</u>

(2) XZ-C4 can inhibit cancer progression and metastasis

In the process of proliferation, cancer cells acquire the malignant nature of infiltration and metastasis. This phenomenon is called the **progression of malignancy**. Research on cancer progression requires reproducible animal models. Therefore, the regressive cancer cell QR-32 isolated from mouse fibrosarcoma was made into this reproducible model. Even if QR-32 is implanted subcutaneously in mice, it will not proliferate, but will completely disappear on its own; if it is injected into a vein, there will be no metastatic nodules in the lungs. However, if gelatin sponge, which is a foreign body in the body, and QR-32 are implanted under the skin of mice, QR-32 will become proliferative cancer cell QRSPO in vivo.

(3) XZ-C1 + XZ-C4 immune regulation and control anti-cancer Chinese medicine

XZ-C1+XZ-C4 immune regulation and control anti-cancer Chinese medicine has the following characteristics:

① Comprehensively improve the quality of life of patients with advanced cancer.

② Protect thymus, improve immunity, protect bone marrow, enhance hematopoietic function, improve immunity and control ability.

③ Enhance physical fitness, relieve pain and improve appetite.

④ Enhance the treatment effect and reduce the side effects of chemotherapy (Figure as the following)

XZ-C1 "Smart Anti-Cancer"

Pharmacodynamics:

96%-100% inhibits cancer cells and has no effect on normal cells.

Pharmacology:

It strengthens the body rightness and protects the positives, dispels the evil without hurting the body, has a strong inhibition on cancer cells, and does not inhibit normal cells.

Toxicology:

Acute toxicity experiments show that there are no obvious side effects and the LD50 is difficult to make. It is a fairly safe prescription.

XZ-C4 "Protector of Thymus and Increase of immune function, Ai-Kang -San"

Pharmacodynamics:

Anti-tumor effect on H22 mice bearing liver cancer:

The tumor inhibition rate of XZ-C4 in the second week was 55%

The tumor inhibition rate of XZ-C4 in the 4th week was 68%

The tumor inhibition rate of XZ-C4 in the 6th week was 70%

Pharmacology:

Promote lymphocyte transformation, enhance cellular immune function, increase white blood cells, inhibit cancer cells, protect immune organs, protect the thymus from atrophy, and protect the breast.

Toxicology:

XZ-C4 can be taken for a long time. Acute toxicity experiments show that the LD50 cannot be produced. It is a safe prescription. Some patients take it for 3-5 years, even 8-10 years, to maintain the body's immunity and prevent cancer recurrence and metastasis. This prescription can be taken orally for a long time and is quite safe and effective anti-cancer and anti-metastasis oral medicine.

16

The experiment and clinical efficacy of XZ-C immune regulation and control anti-cancer Chinese medicine

(1) Anti-tumor effect of XZ-C1+4 anti-cancer Chinese medicine on liver cancer H22 tumor-bearing mice

It was found that H22 tumor-bearing mice were treated for 2 weeks, 4 weeks, and 6 weeks after observation. The tumor inhibition rate increased with the prolonged medication time. The tumor inhibition rate of XZ-C4 was as high as 70% at the 6th week.

After two subsequent repeated tests, the results were stable, indicating that the anti-tumor effect of traditional Chinese medicine was slowly and gradually increased, that is, *the anti-tumor effect was positively correlated with the cumulative dose of traditional Chinese medicine.*

The effect of XZ-C1 and XZ-C4 anti-cancer Chinese medicine on the survival time of H22 tumor-bearing mice:

Experimental results prove that XZ-C1, XZ-C4 anti-cancer Chinese medicine can significantly prolong the survival time of tumor-bearing mice, especially XZ-C4, which significantly prolongs **its survival time** by more than 200%. Not only that, XZ-C4 can also significantly improve the **body Immune function, protection of immune organs, protection of bone marrow, alleviation of side effects of chemotherapy and radiotherapy drugs, no side effects have been seen by mice for 12 months. The above experimental research provides a beneficial basis for clinical application.**

(2) Clinical efficacy

On the basis of experimental research, it has been applied to various types of clinical cancers since 1994, most of which are patients with stage III and IV or above, namely:

1. *Advanced cancer that cannot be removed by exploratory surgery;*

2. *Advanced cancer has lost the indication for surgery;*

3. *Short-term or long-term metastasis or recurrence after various cancer operations;*

4. *Liver metastasis, lung metastasis, brain metastasis of various advanced cancers, or combined with cancerous pleural effusion and cancerous ascites;*

5. *All kinds of cancer resection surgery with estimated interest, exploration can only do gastrointestinal anastomosis or colostomy but not resection;*

6. *Patients who are not suitable for surgery, radiotherapy, chemotherapy, etc.*

XZ-C1, XZ-C4 anti-cancer Chinese medicine has been clinically used for 25 years, and systematically observed, **it has achieved obvious curative effect, and no side effects have been seen after long-term use**. *Clinical observations have proved that XZ-C1, XZ-C4 anti-cancer Chinese medicine can comprehensively improve the quality of life of patients with advanced cancer, improve overall immunity, control cancer cell proliferation, and consolidate and enhance long-term efficacy.*

Oral and external application of XZ-C medicine has a good effect on softening and shrinking metastatic tumors on the body. With intervention or intubation drug pump treatment, it can protect the liver, kidney, bone marrow hematopoietic system and immune organs, and improve immunity.

(3) XZ-C Anticancer Analgesic Ointment has good analgesic effect

Pain is a more obvious and painful symptom for patients with advanced cancer. General analgesics have little effect on cancer pain. Narcotic analgesics are addictive and dependent. *XZ-C Anticancer Analgesic Ointment has strong analgesic effect and lasts for a long time. After 298 cases of clinical verification, the obvious effective rate is 78.0%, and the total effective rate is 95.3%. Repeated use has no obvious side effects, no addiction, and stable pain relief. It is an effective treatment method for cancer patients to relieve pain and improve the quality of life.*

Through experimental research and clinical verification, our experience is:

Traditional Chinese medicine with Chinese characteristics has its unique advantages in tumor treatment, such as strong overall concept, outstanding conditioning effect, mild side effects, can alleviate pain, relieve symptoms, significantly improve the quality of life of patients, and can regulate body immune function and overall resistance. Disease ability and improve treatment effect.

<u>The experimental and clinical observation of XZ-C immunomodulatory anti-cancer traditional Chinese medicine in the treatment of malignant tumors</u>

(1) Experimental results

① The anti-tumor effect of XZ-C Chinese medicine on H22 mice bearing liver cancer:

The tumor inhibition rate of XZ-C1 was 40% in the second week, 45% in the fourth week, and 58% in the sixth week.

The tumor inhibition rate of XZ-C4 in the second week was 55%, the tumor inhibition rate in the fourth week was 68%, and the tumor inhibition rate in the sixth week was 70% 0 (P<0.01)

In the second week of CTX medication, the tumor inhibition rate was 45%. The tumor inhibition rate was 45% in the 4th week, and 49% in the 6th week (Figure 1, Figure 2).

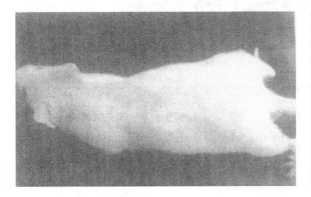
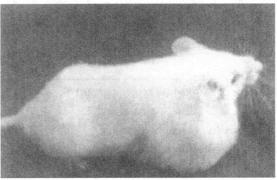

Figure 1 XZ-C1, XZ-C4 treatment group	Figure 2 Control group
30 days after inoculation of liver cancer H22	30 days after inoculation of liver cancer H22

② The effect of XZ-C Chinese medicine on the survival time of H22 mice bearing liver cancer

The average survival days of XZ-C1, XZ-C4 and CTX groups were higher than those of the normal saline control group ((P<0.01); XZ-C Chinese medicine has the effect of prolonging survival period significantly.

Compared with the control group, the life extension rate of XZ-C1 group was 85%, the life extension rate of Z-C4 group was 200%, and the life extension rate of CTX group was 9.8%.

Both XZ-C1 and CTX groups in group B died within 75 days. <u>In XZ-C4 group, 6 cancer-bearing mice were still alive after 7 months.</u>

③ XZ-C1 and XZ-C4 Chinese medicines both increase immune function. XZ-C4 can significantly improve immune function, increase white blood cells and red blood cells, **<u>has no effect on liver and kidney function, and has no damage to liver and kidney slices. CTX reduces white blood cells and reduces immune function. Kidney slices have kidney damage. The thymus in the control group was significantly atrophy</u>** (Figure 3). The thymus in the XZ-C1 and XZ-C4 treatment groups did not shrink and was slightly enlarged (Figure 4).

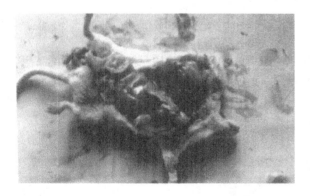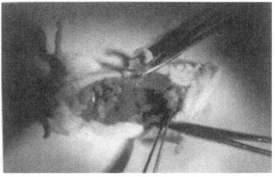

Figure 3 XZ-C4 treatment group	Figure 4 Control group
Thymus hypertrophy 30 days after inoculation with H22	Thymus glands were significantly atrophy 30 days after inoculation with liver cancer H22

Pathological section of control thymus:

The thymic cortex is atrophy, the cells are sparse, and the blood vessels are congested (Figure 5).

Pathological section of thymus in XZ-C4 treatment group:

It shows that the thymic cortex area is thickened, lymphocytes are dense, epithelial reticulocytes increase, and thymic corpuscles increase (Figure 6).

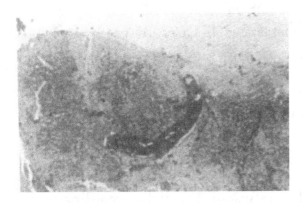 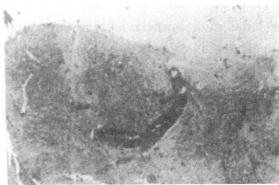

Figure 5 Pathological section of thymus in tumor-bearing control group HEX 100 cortical atrophy The lymphocytes are significantly reduced, a lymphocyte empty zone is formed in the cortex, and intravascular congestion	Figure 6 Thymus in XZ-C4 treatment group HEX 100 Thymus cortical medulla is thickened and lymphocytes are highly dense

(2) Clinical application observation

Clinical information

In Integrated Chinese and Western Medicine Anticancer Research National Collaborative Group Hubei Group, Anti-cancer Metastasis and Recurrence Research Laboratory and Shuguang Oncology Specialist Outpatient Department, from 1994 to November 2002, XZ-C immunomodulation anti-cancer Chinese medicine combined Chinese and Western medicine were used to treat 4698 cases of stage III, IV or metastatic and recurrent cancer, including 3051 males and 1647 females. The youngest is 11 years old, the oldest is 86 years old, and the age at high incidence is 40-69 years old. All patients in the whole group were diagnosed by histopathological diagnosis or B-ultrasound and CL MRI imaging. According to the International Anti-Cancer Alliance's staging standards, all cases are patients with stage III or above in the advanced stage. There are 1021 cases of liver cancer in this group, including 694 cases of primary liver cancer and 327 cases of metastatic liver cancer; 752 cases of lung cancer, including 699 cases of primary lung cancer, 53 cases of metastatic lung cancer; 668 cases of gastric cancer, 624 cases of esophagus and cardia cancer, 328 cases of rectal and anal canal cancer, 442 cases of colon cancer, 368 cases of breast cancer, 74 cases of pancreatic cancer, 30 cases of bile duct cancer, 43 cases of retroperitoneal tumors, 38 cases of ovarian cancer, 9 cases of cervical cancer, 11 cases of brain tumor, 34 cases of thyroid cancer, 38 cases of nasopharyngeal cancer, 9 cases of melanoma, 27 cases of renal cancer, 48 cases of bladder cancer, 13 cases of leukemia, supraclavicular lymph node metastasis 47 cases, 35 cases of various sarcomas, 39 cases of other malignant tumors.

Drugs and methods of administration:

The treatment is to strengthen the body and remove the pathogenic factors, lighten the firm and hard tissue to disperse the masses, tonic the qi and blood, XZ-C1 is a mixture, 150ml daily, XZ-C4 is a powder (infusion), 10g daily, according to the dialectic of the disease, for solid tumor or for metastatic lumps, take anticancer powder orally and anticancer swelling ointment externally. For those with pain, apply topical anticancer pain relief cream. For jaundice and ascites, add Tuihuang Decoction or Xiaoshui Decoction.

Efficacy evaluation:

Not only pay attention to short-term efficacy and imaging indicators, but also pay more attention to long-term efficacy, survival, quality of life and immune indicators. Pay attention to the changes in the subjective symptoms during the medication. If the subjective symptoms improve and last for more than 1 month, it is effective, otherwise it is invalid. The improvement of the quality of life (Kafler score) must be effective for more than 1 month, otherwise it is invalid. The evaluation criteria for the efficacy of solid tumor masses are divided into 4 levels according to the changes in tumor size:

level I: the mass disappears;
level II: the mass is reduced by 1/2;
level III: the mass becomes soft;
level IV: the liver mass is unchanged or enlarged.

Treatment effect

1. Symptoms improved, quality of life improved, and survival time extended:

Among the 4277 patients with intermediate and advanced cancer who took XZ-C immunoregulatory Chinese medicine for more than 3 months, the medical records have detailed curative effect observation records. The overall quality of life of patients has been improved, see Table as the following:

Table Observation of 4277 cases of curative effect, comprehensively improving the quality of life of patients with advanced cancer

Improvement	spirit	Appetite	Strengthen	Generally things get better	Weight gain	Sleep better	Improve activity, ability and vitality, alleviate limitation	Take care of your own life and walk as usual	Resume work, engage in light work
Number of cases	4071	3 986	2 450	479	2938	1005	1038	3220	479
(%)	95.2	93.2	57.3	11.2	68.7	23.5	24.3	75.3	11.2

All patients in this group were in the middle and late stages, and all had different degrees of symptom improvement after taking the medicine, with an effective rate of 93.2%. In terms of improving the quality of life (according to the Karnofsky scoring standard), the average score is 50 before medication, and the average is increased to 80 after medication. The patients in this group have metastasis and dysfunction of different tissues and organs above stage III. Past statistics of such patients It is reported that the median survival time is about 6 months.

The longest cases in this group have reached 21 years, and the average survival time of the remaining cases is more than 1 year.

One case of primary liver cancer in the left lobe of the liver, recurred in the right liver after resection, and has been treated with XZ-C medicine for 21 years;

Another case of liver cancer has been taking XZ-C for 20 and a half years;

In 2 cases of liver cancer, there were multiple cancers in the liver. After taking XZ-C for half a year, the cancers completely disappeared after 2 CT re-examinations and had been stable for half a year.

One case of double kidney cancer had extensive metastasis to the abdominal cavity after one side was resected. After taking XZ-C medicine, he had completely returned to work.

Three cases of lung cancer could not be cut through open thoracotomy, and had been taking XZ-C medicine for 3 and a half years.

Two cases of remnant gastric cancer have been taking XZ-C medicine for 8 years.

Three cases of rectal cancer recurrence took XZ-C medicine for 3 years.

One case of breast cancer metastasized to liver and ribs has been taking medicine for 8 years.

One case of bladder cancer recurred after renal cancer surgery and disappeared after taking XZ-C drug for 9 and a half years.

The above cases are all patients in the middle and late stages who cannot undergo surgery, radiotherapy, or chemotherapy. They only take XZ-C drugs and are not treated with other drugs.

So far, I still come to the clinic every month for review and medicine. After long-term medication, the condition is controlled in a stable state, so that the body and the tumor are in a balanced state for a long time, and a better survival with the tumor is obtained, the patient's symptoms are improved, the quality of life is improved, and the survival period is prolonged.

2. **For 84 patients with solid masses and 56 patients with metastatic supraclavicular lymphadenopathy, oral administration of XZ-C series and external application of XZ-C3 anti-cancer softening knot ointment achieved good results, see Table as the following.**

Table 84

Cases of solid masses and 56 cases of metastatic nodules after
external application of XZ-C ointment changes

Number of Cases	Solid mass				Swollen supraclavicular lymph nodes in the neck			
	Disappear	shrink by ½	Soften	no change	Disappear	shrink by ½	Soften	no change
(%)	12	28	32	12	12	22	14	8
	14.2	33.3	38.0	14.2	21.4	39.2	25.0	14.2
Total effective rate (%)	85.7				85.7			

3. **298 cases of cancer pain patients took XZ-C medicine internally and applied XZ-C anticancer analgesic ointment to obtain significant pain relief effects, as shown in Table as the following.**

Table Pain relief after oral administration of XZ-C medicine and external
application of XZ-C anticancer pain relief ointment in 298 patients

Clinical manifestations	Pain			
	Mild relief	Significantly reduced	Disappear	Invalid
Number of cases	52	139	93	14
(%)	17.3	46.8	31.2	4.7
Total effective rate(%)	95.3			

17

XZ-C immune regulation and control anti-cancer Chinese medicine is the achievement or the result of the modernization of traditional Chinese medicine

XZ-C immune regulation and control anti-cancer Chinese medicine is not an empirical formula, nor is it a famous old Chinese medicine formula, but a scientific research result of the combination of Chinese and Western medicine and the modernization of traditional Chinese medicine.

It uses modern medical methods, combined with experimental tumor experimental research methods and modern pharmacology and pharmacodynamic research methods.

After 7 years of more than 4,000 cancer-bearing animal models, 200 commonly used so-called anti-cancer Chinese herbal medicines were screened in batches by animal experiments. In vitro and in vivo tumor-bearing animals were screened by taste, and 48 kinds of Chinese medicines with good anti-cancer effects were screened out.

These 48 kinds of natural medicines are then formed into $XZ-C_{1-10}$, and according to the respiratory system, digestive system, urinary system, gynecology, endocrine system, the production of liver cancer, gastric cancer, intestinal cancer, breast cancer, bladder cancer, and lung cancer animal models, performing in vivo pharmacodynamic and toxicological experiments in tumor-bearing animals, then they are made into the series of immune regulation and control anti-cancer Chinese medication XZ-C1, XZ-C2, XZ-C3, XZ-C4, XZ-C5, XZ-C6, XZ-C7, XZ-C8, and others.

The material basis for traditional prescriptions to exert their unique curative effect in clinical practice is the chemical components in them. The quality and quantity of chemical constituents are changed, which directly affect the clinical curative effect of prescriptions.

Therefore, only by studying the changes in the quality and quantity of the chemical components in the prescriptions, clarifying the main active ingredients of the preparations, and exploring the mystery of its unique curative effect from the perspective of molecular immunology, it can make the research on traditional prescriptions reach a new level.

The XZ-C immune-regulating Chinese medicine preparation is an innovation and reform of Chinese medicine preparations. It is not a compound liquid of mixed decoction, but a granular concentrate or powder of each medicine. Each crude medicine in each medicine still maintains its original ingredients. The function, molecular weight, and structural formula remain unchanged. It is made by modern scientific methods, not compounding. It keeps the original ingredients and functions of each flavor unchanged, which is convenient for evaluation and affirms the role and curative effect of the medicine.

Facing the future of medicine, looking forward, after 20 years of hard work, practicing the scientific development concept, facing the frontiers of science, and striving for innovation and progress.

To conquer cancer, it must come from the clinic, go through experimental research, and go to the clinic to solve the actual problems of patients; it must seek truth from facts, speak with facts and data; it must constantly surpass ourselves and advance ourselves; in scientific research, it must liberate our minds. Breaking away traditional old concepts, based on independent innovation, and original innovation; our scientific research line for several years is to discover the problem, raise the problem and then research the problem, solve the problem or explain the problem.

The road is like this, step by step, difficult journey, we hope walking on an innovative path of anti-cancer and anti-metastasis with Chinese characteristics and independent intellectual property rights.

Our medical oncology research model is patient-centered, discovering and asking questions from clinical work, conducting in-depth basic research on animal experiments, and then turning the results of basic research into clinical applications to improve the overall level of medical care and ultimately benefit patients.

The pictures as the following:

1. Thymus Atrophy of Cancer-bearing Mouse

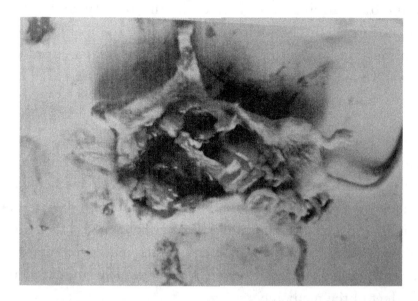

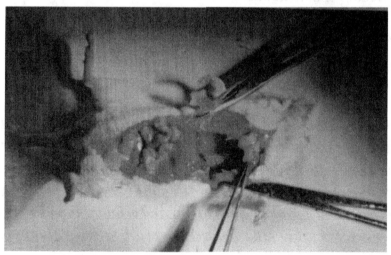

The experimental surgery plays a very important role in developing the medical science and it is one key to open up the out-of-bounds area of the medical science.

The preventive and curing ways of many diseases are applied to the clinic and promote the development of the medical science only when the stable achievements have been made through the experimental research on animals for many times.

2. The animal models for the experimental research on anti-cancer metastasis and recurrence:

1). In an animal model of cancer-bearing animal model, there is a cancerous block which was exfoliative as a whole. The tumor lump completely dropped off from the mouse.

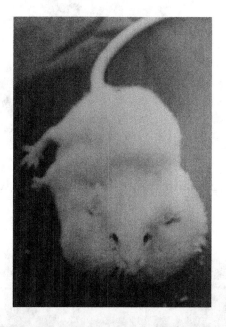

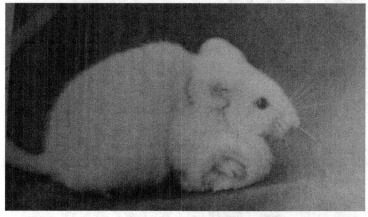

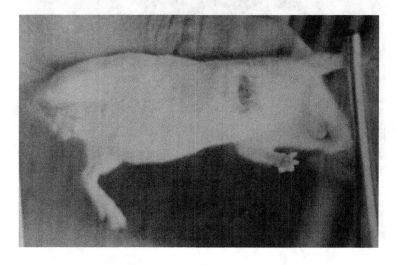

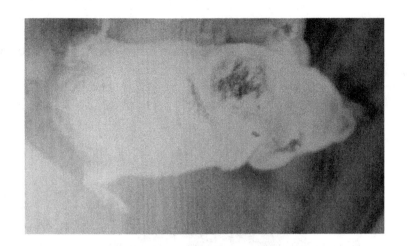

2. ATCA treated S180 sarcoma in tumor-bearing group with S180 sarcoma

The different groups:

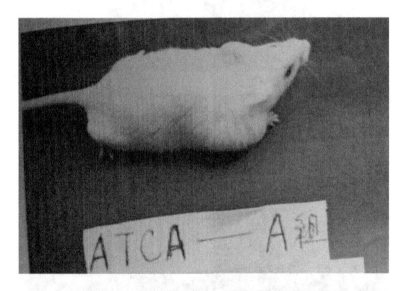

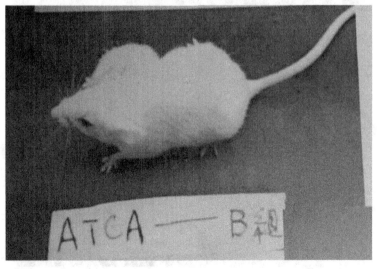

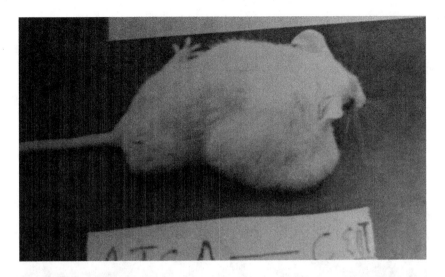

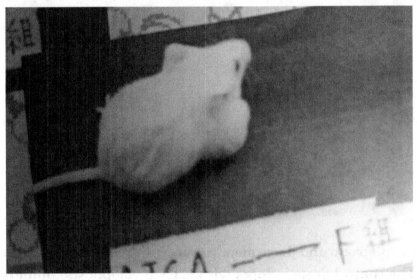

3. XZ-C immune control and regulation medication

The experimental research on protection of Thymus and increase of immune function, protection of bone marrow to produce blood:

Control group and Treatment group with XZ-Cl medication

The control group adopts with CTX (cyclophosphamide)

15 days

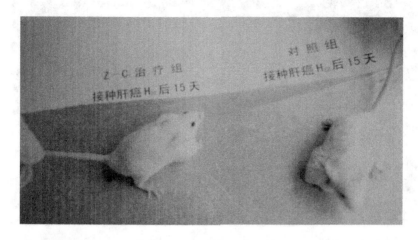

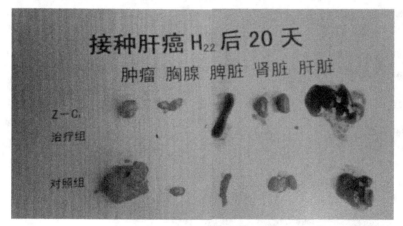

Control group and Treatment group with XZ-C4 medication
The control group adopts with CTX (cyclophosphamide)

20 days

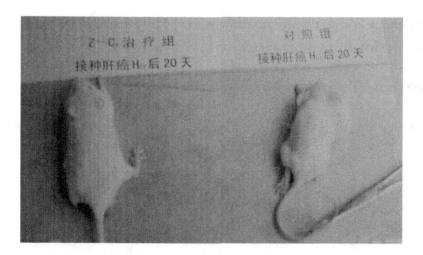

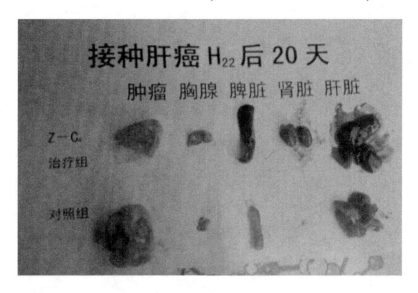

Control group and Treatment group with XZ-C5 medication
The control group adopts with CTX (cyclophosphamide)

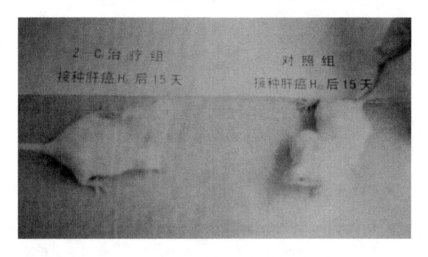

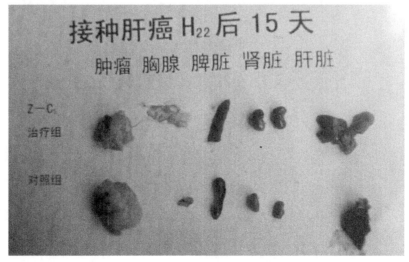

Part IV

The scientific and technological innovation
The scientific and research achievement

Walked out the new way to conquer cancer

1. XZ-C immunomodulatory anti-cancer treatment has been formed

2. For more than 20 years or over the past 20 years, the new path to conquer cancer has been walked out

TABLE OF CONTENTS

Foreword 79

1. The theoretical system of XZ-C immunomodulation for cancer
   treatment has been formed and been undergoing clinical application,
   observation and verification 83
   (1) The Concept of Cancer Therapy.. 83
   (2) Causes and pathogenesis of cancer 89
   (3) Theoretical basis and experimental foundation of cancer treatment....... 97
   (4) Principles of cancer treatment.. 106
   (5) Cancer treatment mode 118
   (6) The principles of cancer metastasis treatment................... 132
   (7) The new concept of cancer metastasis treatment 138
   (8) How to do anti-cancer metastasis? 149
   (9) The methods and drugs of Cancer Treatment.................... 158
   (10) Immunopharmacology of XZ-C immunomodulation anti-Chinese
        medication.. 200

2. This book preliminarily proposes a new concept of XZ-C cancer
   treatment on cancer therapy and analyzes and compares it with
   traditional therapies. It is analyzed with the following table: 203

3. The exclusive scientific research products have been developed 205

4. A large number of clinical cases have been verified XZ-C immune
   regulation and control anti-cancer Chinese medication......................... 207

5. What are the reforms in the book? What are the innovations? 210

6. Research Theoretical Innovation Content of new concepts and new
   methods of cancer metastasis treatment 219

7. Briefly describe the scientific research process of anti-cancer research......... 242

8. Briefly describe the results of anti-cancer research and scientific
   researches(about Dr. Xu Ze and Dr. Bin Wu) 259

9. Accessories 267

FOREWORD

Why was the title of this chapter named as: "Walked out of a New Way to Conquer Cancer"? Or why was the title of the chapter given: "A New Way to Conquer Cancer"?

The origin of the title is due to the guidance and enlightenment in letters from several experts, scholars, predecessors, and teachers:

In the letter from Academician Wu Min dated July 2, 2001:

"The general impression is:

The model from clinical to experimental, and from experimental to clinical is very good. It is also very correct to take the path of combining Chinese and Western medicine. I sincerely hope that you will continue to advance and find a new way to overcome cancer."

Academician Tang Zhaoxian's letter on February 22, 2006 mentioned:

"...Traditional Chinese medicine and biological therapy are the two most promising ways of anti-metastasis, especially Chinese medicine and traditional Chinese medicine. I hope you will take the path of anti-metastasis with Chinese characteristics."

Academician Liu Yunyi's letter on March 22, 2006 mentioned:

"...I very much agree with the concepts and thinking you put forward in the book to conquer cancer. I hope you can make breakthrough contributions in Chinese medicine and traditional Chinese medicine, so that the majority of patients can benefit, so that **Chinese medicine** can be further developed, so that make my country's medical industry reach the world status."

On January 9, 2006, Academician Wu Xianzhong mentioned: "...**Tumors are hard bones to gnaw, but they should continue to gnaw. Fortunately, everyone is very**

objective. As long as it is effective, it will be supported whether it is treating tumors, the body, or alleviating radiological reactions and chemotherapy or chemical reactions. "It also mentioned in the letter dated April 10, 2012: "...I think **the path you have traveled is very unique**. Chinese medicine has innovations in applied dosage forms, administration methods, drug combinations, and the development of XZ-C series of drugs, and has formed its own patent. **This road should continue to be followed and going on.**"

Thank them for their guidance, guidance, and help to our scientific research work, scientific thinking, research direction, research route, research goal, and research method. Our research work has been following the direction of its guidance, and I would like to extend my gratitude to academicians such as Wu Min, Tang Zhaota, Wu Xianzhong, and Liu Yunyi.

In the past 28 years (from 1985 to now), our cancer research work has achieved a series of scientific and technological innovations and scientific research results in animal experimental research, clinical basic research, and clinical verification. After 20 years of hard work, the XZ-C immune control anti-cancer treatment has been formed. In the past 20 years, a new way to conquer cancer has been found.

Over the past 20 years, this series of experimental and clinical research work has been enthusiastically supported and cordially guided by Qiu Fazu, an internationally renowned foreign scientist and a master of general surgery in my country.

In 1990, when Dr. Xu r submitted to the National Science and Technology Commission an application for the "Eighth Five-Year" key scientific and technological project (further explore the anti-cancer and anti-metastasis experimental and clinical research of anti-cancer and anti-cancer Chinese herbal medicine on liver cancer and gastrointestinal cancer precancerous lesions), Academician Qiu stated in the expert opinion:

"Research on cancer metastasis and how to prevent it is a very important topic at present. It is feasible to explore clinical prevention and treatment methods through experimental research, and it is a work that benefits the people."

Under the guidance and guidance of my teacher Qiu Yuan's ten rigorous and scientific style of study, we have initially completed the above project work, and I would like to express my sincere thanks.

Scientific research must be fed by literature.

In 1986, when we had just established an experimental surgical animal laboratory to create animal models of cancer metastasis and conduct experimental research, we saw Professor Gao Jin's book "Cancer Invasion and Metastasis------Basic Research and Clinical ", and read the monograph "Basic and Clinical of Liver Cancer Metastasis and Recurrence" by Academician Tang Zhaotan, the theories in these two books made us suddenly enlightened, and also encouraged and promoted our experimental work and clinical verification work from another aspect.

Professor Tang Zhaotao puts forward in his monograph: ***"The next important goal of primary liver cancer research -------- Prevention* and treatment of recurrence and metastasis**" and said:

"Metastasis and recurrence has become a bottleneck to further improve the survival rate of liver cancer, and it is also one of the most important difficulties in conquering cancer." These theoretical documents have given us the wisdom and courage to update our thinking and be creative, and also strengthen the confidence and determination of our experimental team. I would like to express my gratitude to Academician Tang Zhaotan and Professor Gao Jin.

During 7 years, we had used more than 6000 tumor-bearing animal models to explore basic questions one after another.

In vivo anti-tumor experiment screening of 200 kinds of Chinese herbal medicines in tumor-bearing animal models was completed by several graduate students of mine, including Master Zhu Siping, Dr. Zou Shaomin, Master Li Zhengxun, Master Liu Liling, etc. They carried out and completed a large number of arduous and meticulous experimental work. They worked hard, day and night, and made contributions to the development of anti-cancer and anti-cancer experimental oncology medicine. We would like to express my sincere thanks.

Part IV

Walked out the new way to conquer cancer

XZ-C immunomodulatory anti-cancer treatment has been formed
Over the past 60 years, the new path to conquer cancer has been walked out

1

The theoretical system of XZ-C immunomodulation for cancer treatment has been formed and been undergoing clinical application, observation and verification

(1). The Concept of Cancer Therapy

(Introduction)

1)). The new model of cancer believes_that the **cancer cure should be through regulation and control rather than killing.** The final step in curing cancer is to mobilize or to muster ***the reproduction of the host's control and regulation,*** rather than destroy the last cancer cell. Or,

The new model of cancer considers:

Cure should be through regulation and control rather than killing.

The last step in curing cancer is to mobilize the reappearance of the host's control, rather than destroy the last cancer cells.

2)). The traditional concept is that cancer is the continuous division and proliferation of cancer cells, and its treatment goal must be to kill cancer cells. Therefore, the traditional therapeutic concept of cancer is based on the killing of cancer cells. In order to achieve cure, the last cancer cell must be killed, so people have used expanded surgery, intensified chemotherapy and radical radiotherapy, but the results are not satisfactory.

Quoted the original article in Chapter 1 from "Monograph"

(1) The concept of cancer therapy

(The description of the brief introduction)

1). <u>The new concept for cancer treatment</u>
2). Traditional therapeutic concepts of cancer

1). The new concept of cancer treatment

<u>The cancer cure should be through regulation and control rather than killing</u>

<u>Healing should be through regulation and control rather than killing</u>

Why is this new concept proposed? What will be the reasons for this new concept?

The leading or guidance ideas of the new cancer model are:

The regulation and signal transmission between cells in cancer patients are *<u>disrupted</u>* rather than lost; the carcinogenesis is considered to be a *<u>continuum with the possibility of reversal</u>*. **Or** it is considered that carcinogenesis is a continuum with the **possibility of reversal**.

<u>The understanding of cancer in the new model is based on information transmission and regulatory control.</u>

*It recognizes that malignant transformation is **a gradually progressiving process, but also believes that they have the potential to reverse.***

<u>The new model of cancer therapy believes that the cancer cure should be through regulation and control rather than killing.</u>

The experience of clinical practice and experimental research reminds us: *<u>there is a certain response relationship between the tumor and the host.</u>*

If the tumor is regarded as the result of an imbalance in regulation and control, rather than the autonomous behavior of the tumor, some clinical phenomena are easier to understand.

We know that clinically tumor cells can make a highly adaptive response to the host environment.

For example:

1. Long-term application of immunosuppressive drugs can induce tumors.

When the immunosuppressive drugs are stopped, the tumors can be completely relieved.

Although the factors that induce tumors have not been confirmed, the host's response determines the final result.

2. Renal tumors with existing lung metastases can be completely relieved after stopping anti-rejection therapy.

3. Pregnancy also seems to change the relationship between the tumor and the host.

Turning our attention to the killing of tumors, for half a century, people have developed a variety of treatment methods and developed many anti-cancer drugs, but they still have not stopped the invasion and metastasis of tumors.

From the current data, adjuvant chemotherapy with cytotoxic drugs after surgery has failed to prevent the recurrence and metastasis of cancer.

It is because most of them will have a severe inhibitory effect on immune function, and it can even suppress the host response from the non-immune part. When we perform intensive chemotherapy, it is likely to cause artificial or iatrogenic immune failure.

At present, from a molecular biology perspective, cancer is a change in the DNA structure of a cell, a disorder of cell differentiation caused by a change in genetic information. The introduction of normal nucleic acids into tumor cells through genetic engineering can induce tumor cells to differentiate into normal paper cells. The Shanghai Cancer Institute once extracted ribonucleic acid from normal hepatocytes and incubated with hepatocytes to culture. Through the regulation and control of normal hepatic ribonucleic acid and other regulatory functions, the abnormal gene activity of liver cancer cells was corrected, which led to the reversal to the normal cells.

Science is looking for living active substances related to genetic information, such as normal information ribonucleic acid (mRNA) can induce cancer cells to reverse to normal cells.

The use of cytotoxic drugs to treat cancer is based on the premise that the last cancer cell must be killed until the tumor has been completely eliminated in the clinical and laboratory.

But based on our 60 years of experience, there are still many contradictions in this view. Some clinical examples show that the use of killing can shrink or regress the tumor, but it is not necessarily a direct cure.

As the amount of cytotoxic drugs continues to increase, most patients' cancer cells begin to subside, but the patient's survival rate has not improved, and will soon relapse and the tumor will increase.

It seems that patients who have been cured obviously did not use cell killing methods.

For example,

1, ***the treatment of tumors with platinum drugs seems to be related to the induction of cell differentiation.***

2, *the effects of **interferon and interleukin** on sensitive cells also play a role through regulatory control mechanisms.*

3, *as an adjunct therapy for colorectal cancer, **levamibia is** believed to have an effect from changes in host auto-response.*

In the past, it has tried the best to treat cancer cells, but they have not been very successful. People adopted expanded radical cure, intensive chemotherapy and radical radiotherapy. However, the results were not satisfactory and did not improve the quality of life of cancer patients and prolong the survival time of cancer patients.

In the past 60 years, Chinese medicine has made great achievements in the treatment of cancer. *A large amount of data reported everywhere indicates that cancer cells can coexist with the host, and the host has a long survival time.*

In the past several years, among the more than 12,000 patients with advanced cancer in the Shuguang Cancer Institute and Wuchang Shuguang Oncology Specialty

Clinic, some were relapsed and metastatic patients, such as recurrent cancer at the anastomosis and gastric cancer, and those who could not be removed and could not do radiotherapy or chemotherapy. For these patients, after the long-term administration of XZ-C immunomodulatory Chinese medicine for 3-5 years, their condition is controlled, the patients survive stably (coexist with cancer), the life is completely self-care, the quality of life is good, and the survival period is significantly prolonged.

*We believe that dealing with outsiders who invade the body should undoubtedly be mercilessly killed. However, for treating cancer cells it is different to some degree, because they are only mutated tissues in the normal body of the host itself, so cancer should be controlled and regulated by **adjusting the body**. But It is not necessary and also impossible to kill all cancer cells.*

With a new understanding of the concept of cancer, the concept of cancer therapy should also update ideas and knowledge, and then innovate treatment theories and technologies.

In view of our experience and lessons in more than the past half century, it should find *a breakthrough in clinical research* from the current urgent problems of cancer research and the weakness of modern medicine, and find a breakthrough in *prevention and treatment* from the aspects of invasion, recurrence and metastasis; it is looking for the *effective anti-relapse and anti-metastatic drugs from chemical synthetic drugs and natural drugs*. *Targeted treatment* is carried out from the molecular level, gene level, and comprehensive treatment level to deepen the new understanding of the concept of cancer.

2). Traditional therapeutic concepts of cancer

Traditional therapeutic concepts believe that cancer is the continuous division and proliferation of cancer cells, and its treatment goal must be to kill cancer cells. Therefore, the goals of the three traditional treatments are all based on killing cancer cells.

The basic principle of traditional cancer treatment is that the last cancer cell must be killed or eliminated. Therefore, people have adopted expanded surgery, intensive chemotherapy and radical radiotherapy. But the result is not satisfactory.

In the early 1960s, the scope of oncology surgery tended to expand, and a series of super radical operations were developed. **After years of practice, it has been proved that expanding the scope of surgical resection, such as breast cancer, lung cancer,**

liver cancer, and pancreatic cancer, has not changed the cancer-free survival and overall survival of patients.

In the 1980s, intensive chemotherapy and radical radiotherapy failed to improve the quality of life or prolong the survival period. Instead, due to the severe suppression of bone marrow hematopoietic function and immune function, some life-threatening complications were added. This reminds us that it may be necessary to establish a new model, try to explore from other angles, update ideas, and open up new paths.

In short, the traditional concept believes that cancer is based on crazy cell division and proliferation, and cancer cells are the culprit. Therefore, in traditional cancer therapy, the target of treatment is set to cancer cells, and the goal is to kill cancer cells.

"Monogram"-" New Concepts and Methods of Cancer Treatment" (the third monograph version)

(2). The etiology or causes and pathogenesis of cancer

(Brief Introduction)

In order to explore the ***etiology, pathogenesis, and pathophysiology*** of cancer, a series of animal experimental studies was conducted.

The new discoveries, new thinking, and new enlightenment are obtained after we analyzed and though over the experimental results as the followings:

Atrophy of the thymus and low immune function are one of the causes and pathogenesis of cancer.

Therefore, at the international conference Professor XU ZE proposed that **one of the causes and pathogenesis of cancer may be atrophy of the thymus, impaired function of central immune organs, weakened immune function, decreased ability of immune surveillance and immune escape.**

After checking for novelty, this is the first time it has been proposed internationally. (See Chapter 2 of this book)

Quote from the original article in my monograph in Chapter 2

(2) Causes and pathogenesis of cancer

Atrophy of thymus and low immune function may be one of the causes or etiology and pathogenesis of cancer

(The description of brief Introduction)

1). The new findings in experimental research on cancer etiology, pathogenesis and pathophysiology

2). It is to explore methods to curb tumor progression and progressive thymus atrophy and to reconstruct immune function

1). The new findings in experimental research on the cause, pathogenesis and pathophysiology of cancer

In the past many years, we have carried out a series of experimental studies on animal experiments to explore *the possible causes, pathogenesis, and pathophysiology of cancer,* explore *the mechanisms of cancer invasion, recurrence, and metastasis*, and search *the effective measures for regulation and control.*

The experimental surgery is extremely important in the development of medical science. It is a key to open the medical restricted area. Many disease prevention and treatment methods are applied to the clinic after many animal experimental studies have achieved stability results.

Therefore, Dr. Xu Ze established an experimental surgery laboratory to conduct the experimental tumor research, perform cancer cell transplantation, establish a tumor animal model, and carried out the following series of experimental tumor research:

①. *To explore the experimental research on the etiology, pathogenesis and pathophysiology of cancer;*

②. *To explore the mechanism and regularity or rules of cancer recurrence and metastasis;*

③. *To explore the relationship between tumor and immune and immune organs, and between immune organs and tumors;*

④. *To explore methods to curb tumor progression and progressive atrophy of immune organs and to reconstruct immune function;*

⑤. *To look for effective measures to regulate and to control cancer invasion, recurrence and metastasis.*

From the experimental tumor research it was found that, in order to explore the etiology, pathogenesis, invasion and metastasis mechanisms of cancer, and to find effective measures for regulation and control, intervention, recurrence, and metastasis, the author and colleagues conducted a full four years of experimental tumor research. Some of the experimental results are as the followings:

(1) *Experiment 1:*

Removal of mouse thymus ((Thyinus, TH) creates cancer-bearing animal models, or injection of immunosuppressive drugs helps to establish cancer-bearing animal models.

The conclusion of the study proves that the occurrence and development of cancer is significantly related to the host immune organ thymus and its function relationship.

(2) Experiment 2:

Whether is it immune decreasing first and then easy to get cancer, or cancer occur first and then immune weak?

The experimental results confirm:

Immune function is low first and then cancer is prone to develop. If there is no decline in immune function, cancer inoculation is not easy to succeed.

The results of the experiment suggest that improving and maintaining good immune function and protecting the good central immune organ thymus are one of the important measures to prevent cancer.

(3) Experiment 3:

When studying the relationship between cancer metastasis and immune function, an animal model of liver metastatic cancer was established and divided into two groups, A and B. Immunosuppressive drugs were used in group A and not in group B.

The result is:

The number of intrahepatic metastases in group A was significantly higher than that in group B.

Tips of the experiment results:

Metastasis is related to immune function. Immune function or application of immunosuppressive drugs may promote tumor metastasis.

(4) Experiment 4:

When exploring the effect of tumors on the body's immune organs, it was found that as the cancer progresses, the thymus is progressively atrophied. The host's thymus is acutely atrophied after inoculating tumor cells, cell proliferation is blocked, and the volume is significantly reduced.

The experimental results suggest that the tumor may suppress the thymus and cause the immune organs to shrink.

(5) Experiment 5:

In the experiment, it was found that in some experimental mice which cancer cells were not successfully inoculated into or the tumor grew very small, their thymus did not shrink significantly.

In order to understand the relationship between the tumor and thymus atrophy, a group of experimental mice were resectioned or autopsied when the solid tumor grew to the size of the thumb. One month later, anatomy revealed that the thymus did not progressively shrink.

Therefore, we speculate that the solid tumor may produce a factor that is not yet known to suppress the thymus, which needs further experimental research.

(6) Experiment 6:

The above experimental results all prove:

The progress of the tumor can make the thymus progressively shrink, so can some methods be used to prevent the atrophy of the host thymus?

Through animal experiments, we began to find ways or drugs to prevent atrophy of thymus in tumor-bearing mice.

The transplantation of the immune organ cells was used to restore the function of the immune organ, and it was to explore the methods of curbing tumor progression, stopping atrophy of the thymus of the immune organ, and reconstructing immune functions.

The experimental research of that the rats were transplanted with fetal liver, fetal spleen and fetal thymus cells, and adoptive immunity to reconstruct their immune function was done.

The result shows:

In the combined transplantation of S. T. L cells in the three groups, the recent complete tumor regression rate was 40%, and the long-term tumor complete regression rate was 46.67%. Those with complete tumor regression achieved long-term survival.

(7) Experiment 7:

In experiments that explored the effect of tumors on the spleen of the body's immune organs, it was found that:

The spleen has an inhibitory effect on tumor growth in the early stage of the tumor, and in the late stage of the tumor, the spleen also progressively atrophy.

The research results suggest:

The effect of the spleen on tumor growth is bidirectional, with a certain inhibitory effect in the early stage and no inhibitory effect in the late stage. Spleen cell transplantation can enhance the effect of inhibiting tumor.

(8) Experiment 8:

The follow-up results suggest:

Controlling metastasis is the key to cancer treatment.

At present, it is known that there are multiple steps and links in cancer cell metastasis. In order to try to block one of the links to prevent its metastasis, it is believed that tumor neovascularization is one of the steps for whether metastatic cancer cells can implant and take root and become cancerous nodules.

In 1986, Dr. Xu Ze **carried out microcirculation research work**, using microcirculation microscope to observe the microvessel formation and flow velocity of tumor nodules in cancer-bearing mice, and then looked for anti-tumor angiogenesis drugs from natural drugs.

Microcirculation photomicrography system was used to observe the formation process of new microvessels and count the flow rate of arterioles and venules, and *then screened the extract of flavin acid cool acid (TG).*

It turns out:

On the first day of inoculation, there was no neovascularization, and on the second day, the growth of slender neovascularization was seen. TG can reduce the density of new microvessels that enter and exit the tumor.

(9) Experiment 9:

A large number of tumor-bearing animal models in the laboratory have found that *the larger the solid tumors subcutaneously inoculated in some cancer-bearing experimental mice are, the more different the cancer cells in the central tissue structure are from the surrounding cancer cells, and in the nodular centers there are mostly sterile necrosis or liquefaction, in the surrounding areas there are still active cancer cells.*

Therefore, in clinical treatment work, treatment measures for cancer with aseptic necrosis can be taken.

2). **To explore methods to curb cancer progression, progressive atrophy of the thymus, and rebuild immune function**

The above experimental research suggests that one of the etiology and pathogenesis of cancer may be thymus atrophy, thymocyte proliferation is blocked, thymus function is impaired, and immune function is low, leading to immune escape of malignant cells.

Since the thymus will undergo progressive atrophy as the tumor progresses, how can intervention be taken to prevent its atrophy?

Through animal experiment research to look for a way or medicine to prevent thymus atrophy in tumor-bearing mouse, it finally transplanted the immune organ cells to restore the function of these immune organs, and achieved the exciting results.

At that time, we had considered to apply the above experimental methods for clinical trial, trying to use the stillbirth induced by water bladder to take thymus to try to make homogenate allogeneic thymocyte transplantation, but medical ethics was not allowed, so it was not implemented.

In 1986, at a satellite meeting of an international conference on microcirculation, Dr. Xu Ze was inspired by the discussion about looking for microcirculation drugs from natural medicines, changed the research from the biological cell transplantation of adoptive immunity to immune reconstruction to look for the natural medicals, then *turned to search activation Cytokines enhance immune surveillance, thereby suppressing tumors and preventing thymus atrophy from the natural medicines of Chinese herbal medicines.*

All medicines must pass animal experiments and clinical verification, so in the study of cancer-bearing animal models, after more than 3 years, more than 200 flavors were screened for tumor suppression screening from natural medicines and herbs.

In the end, anti-cancer immune-modulating Chinese herbal medicine with good tumor suppressing effect was selected.

Through the experimental screening to clinical observation and verification, then further screening and concentration from traditional Chinese medicine immunopharmacology into XZ-C$_{1-10}$ anti-cancer immune regulation and control traditional Chinese medicine, which can not only promote thymus hyperplasia, prevent thymus atrophy, but also enhance immune function, protect bone marrow, promote T lymphocyte function and cytokines, and has a high tumor suppression rate, only inhibit cancer cells without affecting normal cells, and can be taken orally for a long time.

Because cancer is a chronic disease, the division, proliferation, and cloning of cancer cells are long-term, continuous, and progressive, therefore, it is advisable to choose a long-term, non-toxic, orally-administerable drug.

The treatment of cancer with Chinese herbal medicine is to identify the cause and mechanism of the treatment from the overall point of view of the person. It is not only to kill cancer cells, but also to improve the body's own immune function, thereby enhancing the body's anti-cancer ability, so it can control some refractory and widely metastatic cancers, prolong the lives of cancer patients, and reduce the suffering of patients. It has opened a path worthy of further exploration for cancer treatment.

The results of a series of animal experiments exploring the etiology, pathogenesis, and pathophysiology of cancer have inspired us <u>that thymectomy leads to immunodeficiency, which leads to a decline in immune surveillance and eventually development of immune escape.</u>

This may be one of the keys to the etiology and pathogenesis of cancer. It is a new development of oncology theory in the 21ⁿᵈ century, which provides direction and basis for cancer therapy in the 21ⁿᵈ century, and provides a theoretical basis and experimental basis for cancer immunomodulation targeted therapy.

This innovative discovery has not been mentioned in domestic and foreign textbooks and literature.

Once the above theories and theories have been demonstrated and accepted, they will cause a series of changes and updates in cancer therapeutics, such as:

1. the changes and updates in the understanding of cancer treatment concepts;
2. the changes and updates in the understanding of cancer treatment goals or targets;
3. the changes and updates on cancer diagnosis methods and curative effect judgment standards;
4. the changes and updates on cancer treatment methods and treatment models;
   5.the changes and updates on research and development of anti-cancer and anti-metastatic drugs.

The summary of the course of the research and work is as the followings :

In 1985, I interviewed more than 3,000 patients with chest and abdomen cancer after surgery, and found that:
Recurrence and metastasis are the key factors affecting the long-term postoperative efficacy.

$\downarrow$

How to prevent recurrence and metastasis requires basic clinical research

$\downarrow$

So we established an animal laboratory

↓

Making the cancer-bearing animal model

↓

Our laboratory has the following new findings:

The experimental discovery 1:	The experimental discovery 2:	The experimental discovery 3:	The experimental discovery 4:	The experiment discovery 5:	The experiment discovery 6:
Thymus excision can make animal models of cancer.	Using immunosuppressive drugs to make immune ↓ is conducive to making animal models of cancer.	As the cancer progresses, the thymus progressively shrinks	Cancer metastasis is related to immune function. And low immune function may promote tumor metastasis.	The inoculated mice with cancer had progressive atrophy of the thymus, but the thymus did not atrophy when it was not inoculated with cancer cells. The thymus no longer atrophied when cancer grew to the size of the fingertips and was removed.	The tumor suppresses Thymus (TH) and causes the immune organs to shrink. Therefore, it is deduced that solid tumors may produce a factor that is not yet known to inhibit TH, which is estimated and called "cancer suppressor thymus factor".

↓

The experimental results of our laboratory mentioned above are as the followings:

Tumor progression has the following functions:

1. it can make progressive atrophy of immune organ Thymus.

2. It can make the body's immune function decreasing progressively.

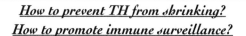

How to prevent TH from shrinking?

How to promote immune surveillance?

Our laboratory conducted the following research work:

How to make Thymus not shrink? *How to make immunity not exhausted?*	*How to stop Thymus from shrinking?* *How to protect immune organs?* *How to avoid immune failure?*
The fetal liver, fetal cell gland, fetal spleen cell transplantation were performed, adoptive immunization which was done to rebuild the immune function.	We look for Chinese medicine resources to prevent thymus atrophy and increase immunity.
The results showed that the combined transplantation of the three groups of S, T, and L cells had a complete tumor regression rate of 40% in the near future and a tumor regression rate of 46.67% in the long-term.	*So the experimental screening from 200 kinds of traditional Chinese medicines was conducted to look for Chinese medicines for Thymus protection, bone marrow protection and blood production, and anti-relapse and transfer.*
The experimental papers cannot be published	*After 3 years of laboratory screening experiments:* *1. Screening experiment of tumor inhibition rate in vitro tube culture:* *2. Screening experiment of tumor inhibition rate in cancer-bearing animal models.*
It is shifted to use traditional Chinese medicine as a resource, which is screened and searched from natural medicine through animal experiments.	

(3)   Theoretical basis and experimental foundation of cancer treatment

(Brief Introduction)

As a result of the laboratory experiments, it was found that:

The thymus of cancer-bearing mice is progressively atrophy, and the central immune organ function is impaired, the immune function is reduced, and the immune surveillance is low, *so the treatment principle must be to prevent the progressive atrophy of the thymus, promote thymus hyperplasia, protect the bone marrow hematopoietic function, improve immunity monitor and control the immune escape of malignant cells.*

Based on the enlightenment of the above experimental research results on cancer etiology and pathogenesis, the new theories and methods of XZ-C immunomodulatory therapy are proposed.

After 60 years of oncology specialist outpatient clinics, more than 12,000 cases of middle- and advanced-stage cancer patients have been clinically observed and confirmed by the author to prove that the treatment principle of Thymus protection and enhancing immunization is reasonable and the efficacy is satisfactory.

XZ-C (XU ZE China) immunomodulation therapy was first proposed by Professor Xu Ze in his book "New Concepts and Methods of Cancer Metastasis Treatment" in 2006.

It is believed that under normal circumstances, the cancer and the body's defenses are in a dynamic balance, and the occurrence of cancer is caused by the imbalance of the dynamic balance. If the disordered state is adjusted to a normal level, the growth of cancer can be controlled and resolved.

As we all know, the occurrence, development and prognosis of cancer are determined by the comparison of two factors, **namely the biological characteristics of cancer cells and the host's own body's ability to restrict and defend cancer cells.**

If the two are balanced, the cancer can be controlled. *Imbalance* between cancer and host's ability to restrict and defend cancer cells is then the development of cancer.

Under normal circumstances, the host's body itself has certain restrictions on cancer cells, **but when the patient is suffering from cancer, these restrictions and defense capabilities are inhibited and damaged to varying degrees, resulting in losing immune surveillance of cancer cells and cancer cells have cellular immune escape, which makes cancer cells further develop and metastasize.**

(See P17 in Chapter 3 of the above book)

Quoted from Chapter 3 of the original "Monograph"

(3) Theoretical basis and experimental foundation for cancer treatment

(Demonstration of Brief introduction)
The theoretical basis and experimental foundation
of XZ-C immunomodulation therapy:

"Protection of Thymus and Enhancing Immune function"

Summary

1). The inspiration from the animal experiment

2). It should protect, regulate and control, and activate the anti-cancer immune system in the human body

3). The overview of research on biomodulator-like immune regulation and control of anti-cancer chinese medicatoin

4). The biological response modifier-like effects and therapeutic effects of XZ-C immunomodulates chinese medication

1). The inspiration of the animal experiment

In the author's laboratory it was found that the thymus glands of cancer-bearing mice were progressively atrophied, and the central immune organs were damaged, <u>so their treatment should be protected by "Thymus protection and increasing immune function" to protect the thymus gland and increase immune function.</u>

<u>Based on the enlightenment of the experimental research results on the etiology and pathogenesis of cancer, Professor Xu Ze first proposed the new theory and method of XZ-C immune regulation and control targeted therapy.</u>

As a result of the experimental research, it was found that all cancer-bearing mice had progressive atrophy of the thymus and impaired central immune organ function, decreased immune function, and low immune surveillance.

Therefore, the treatment principle should be to prevent progressive atrophy of the thymus and promote thymic hyperplasia, protect the bone marrow hematopoietic function, improve immune surveillance, and control the immune escape of malignant cells.

As we all know, there are central immune organs and peripheral immune organs. The former is thymus, bone marrow, and the latter is spleen and lymph nodes etc. It has been confirmed that when cancer occurs, a factor that suppresses immune organs [we will temporarily call it a cancer suppressor Thymus (immuno) factor] suppresses the thymus, causing the thymus to gradually shrink and the function of central immune organs to be suppressed. In turn, the immune function declines, which causes to be weakening or missing immune surveillance, and the tumor must inevitably develop further.

After 16 years of clinical verification and observation of more than 12,000 patients with advanced cancer in the oncology clinic, it has been confirmed that the treatment principle of Thymus protection and enhancing immune function is correct and reasonable, and the effect is satisfactory.

XZ-C (XU ZE-China) immunomodulation therapy was first proposed by Professor Xu Ze of China in 2006 in his book "New Concepts and Methods of Cancer Metastasis Treatment".

It is believed that under normal circumstances, *there is a dynamic balance between cancer and the body's defense, and the occurrence and development of cancer is caused by the imbalance of dynamic balance. If the disordered state is adjusted to a normal level, the growth of cancer can be controlled and resolved*.

As we all know, the occurrence and development of cancer and the prognosis depend on the comparison of two factors, namely the biological characteristics of cancer cells and the host's own body's ability to restrict and defend cancer cells. If the two are balanced, the cancer can be controlled. Imbalance of these Two factors is the development of cancer.

Under normal circumstances, the host's body itself has certain restrictions on cancer cells, but when the patient is suffering from cancer, these restrictions and defense capabilities will be inhibited and damaged to varying degrees, resulting in cancer cells losing immune surveillance and cancer cells. The immune escape makes the cancer cells further develop and metastasize.

2). **It should protect, regulate and control, and activate the anti-cancer immune system in the human body**

When discussing the principles of cancer treatment, it should be studied about which <u>anti-cancer immune cell series</u>, which <u>anti-cancer cytokine series</u>, which

anti-cancer gene series, and which the **humoral immune series** exist in the human body.

1)). <u>What anti-cancer immune cells</u> in the human body may be activated and strengthened to resist cancer cell metastasis?

(A) <u>Cytotoxic lymphocytes (CTL):</u>

    a. It plays a major role in anti-tumor immunity.
    b. Human CTL cells are CD3 and CD8.
    c. CTL cells are high in peripheral blood and spleen, and there are certain contents in thoracic duct, thymus, and bone marrow.
    d. Under certain conditions, it can also produce IL-2, IL-4, INF and other cytokines.
    e. It activates other anti-cancer immune cells and killer macrophages, natural killer cells and killer B cells to play an anti-tumor effect.

(B) <u>Natural killer cells (NK cells):</u>

    a. NK cells are a group of broad-spectrum anti-cancer cells.
    b. Their killing activity is independent of antibodies and thymus.
    c. Their main role is to monitor and eliminate cancerous cells in the body.
    d. Clinical observations have shown that the incidence of malignant tumors is significantly increased in people with defects in NK activity.
    e. NK cells are an important part of the body's early anti-cancer immune surveillance function.

(C) <u>LAK cells:</u>

    a. LAK cells are the most important anti-cancer cells in modern biological therapy.
    b. Human peripheral mononuclear cells (PBMNC) can significantly kill a variety of human tumor cells under the induction of IL-2 in vitro.
    c. LAK cells have a broader tumor killing spectrum than NK cells.
    d. It can also kill tumor cells which NK cells cannot.

(D) <u>Macrophages (Mφ):</u>

It plays an important role in the body's anti-tumor immunity.

2)). What <u>anti-cancer factors</u> in the human body can be activated and enhanced to resist cancer metastasis?

(A) Interferon (IFN):

a. Interferon can resist cell differentiation and has immunoregulatory functions.
b. It has anti-proliferative effect on some tumor cells, and its anti-cancer effect may be related to immune regulation.
c. It can enhance the activity of NK cells and Mφ cells.

(B) Interleukin-2 (IL-2):

It is a T-cell growth factor with strong immunoregulatory functions, which can promote the activation of T cells, NK cells and monocytes, as well as the release of IFN-a and TNF.

(C) Tumor necrosis factor (TNF):

Its effect on cells is cytotoxic, and can affect the microvessels of the tumor, eventually leading to necrosis in the center of the tumor.

(3) Other

In recent years, due to the rapid development of molecular biology, molecular immunology, molecular immunopharmacology, and genetic engineering, the basic and clinical research at the molecular level of "anti-cancer institutions" has been continuously expanded and deepened, and its anti-cancer and anti-metastatic research prospects are very attractive people.

At present, the research on anti-cancer molecular biological immunotherapy mainly focuses on **<u>the four subsystems of anti-cancer institutions, namely anti-cancer cell therapy, anti-cancer cell factor therapy, anti-cancer gene therapy and anti-cancer antibody therapy.</u>**

The basic feature of these molecular biology and molecular immunotherapy is that all the preparations of molecular biological immunotherapy are the organism's own substance, and the fundamental difference between it and radiotherapy and chemotherapy is that *<u>it not only has no progressive damage to the normal tissue cells of the body, especially the cells and functions of the immune system, and the structure and function of the bone marrow hematopoietic system, but also has regulation and enhancement function to immune response.</u>*

As we all know, radiotherapy and chemotherapy are non-selective "damaging therapies" that kill cancer cells as well as normal cells, which will damage the normal tissue cells of the body, causing severe damage to the bone marrow hematopoietic system and immune structure and function, resulting in serious consequences.

Biological therapy is a kind of therapy that stabilizes and balances the life mechanism through the adjustment of biological response. American scholar Oldham put forward the theory of biological regulation in 1984, and then put forward the concept of **tumor biotherapy on this basis.**

3)). *The overview of research on biomodulator-like immune regulation and control of anti-cancer chinese medication*

XZ-C immunomodulated anti-cancer Chinese medicine has been confirmed by animal experiments and clinical practice to have bio-modulator-like effects and curative effects. It is the drug selected from natural medicine resources.

The experimental screening work is mainly carried out through the in vivo tumor suppression experiment of the tumor-bearing animal model.

An experimental group of blind Chinese medication was observed in the animal model for 3 months.

The 48 effective anti-cancer Chinese herbal medicines screened are matched with every 2 flavors or every 3 flavors to perform in vivo tumor inhibition experiments on tumor-bearing animals, it was found that the tumor inhibition experiment of a single chinese medication is not as good as the compound tumor inhibition experiment of an optimized combination of multiple chinese medication, and a single chinese medication only has an inhibitory effect on tumor proliferation. *However, the compound of the optimized combination of multi-flavor Chinese traditional medications not only has an inhibitory effect on the tumor proliferation of tumor-bearing animals, but also has a good regulatory and control effect on the body's immune regulation and control, strengthening physical strength, improving immune function, promoting tumor suppressor cytokine production, and protecting normal cells.*

On the basis of the in vitro experimental screening of single traditional Chinese medicine and the screening of tumor-bearing tumor models in tumor-bearing animal models for 4 years, and then through an optimized combination of experiments, after re-testing, it is reorganized into the compound of XZ-C$_{1-10}$ immunomodulatory anti-cancer, anti-metastatic and anti-relapse. Finally, clinical verification is performed.

Since 1992, Dr. Xu Ze has organized a collaboration group to conduct clinical verification.

After 60 years of clinical verification and observation of more than 12,000 patients with various cancers in the Shuguang Oncology Specialist Clinic, the patients who are treated with these medications have stable and improved conditions, improved symptoms, and improved quality of life. The survival period is obviously extended.

Many patients with metastases stabilized the lesion after taking the drug, and the cancer cells did not spread or metastasize further.

Some patients could not undergo radiotherapy or chemotherapy due to postoperative white blood cell count reduction. After taking the drug, the metastasis was controlled and did not metastasize.

4). *The biological response modifier-like effects and therapeutic effects of XZ-C immunomodulates chinese medication*

The biological response regulation was first described by Oldham in 1982. Its significance is the ability to regulate the body's response or response to external "attacks" through biological response modifiers (BRM).

The cells and humoral factors of the body's immune system are under subtle regulation and control.

In the case of loss of balance, the body's ability to respond or respond will be significantly affected.

The use of biological response modifiers is to restore the state of the body that has lost its balance to the normal state of balance, so as to achieve the prevention and treatment of diseases.

BRM has opened up new areas of cancer biotherapy. At present, BRM is widely regarded as the fourth mode of cancer treatment by the medical community.

The biological response modifier has the function of regulating the body's immune function and restoring the suppressed body's immune system.

Its mechanism of action is multifaceted, but no matter what kind of mechanism, it is through the activation of the body's immune system to exert its regulatory function.

Biological response modifiers are mostly derived from microorganisms and plants. Previously, they were called immunopotentiators, immunostimulants, immune exciting factors, or immunomodulators. They are now collectively named biological response modifiers or modifiers.

Dr. Xu Ze has screened and selected the XZ-C immunomodulatory anti-cancer and anti-metastasis Chinese medicines through the experiments of tumor-bearing mice in vivo, which have a good tumor suppression rate and have improved immunity, protected the central immune organ thymus, improved cellular immunity, and protected thymus tissue function, increasing immunity, protecting bone marrow blood function, increasing red blood cell and white blood cell count, activating immune cytokines, improving immune surveillance in the blood and so on.

The main pharmacological effect of XZ-C immunomodulatory anti-cancer traditional Chinese medicine is "Protection of Thymus and enhancing immune function".

After 60 years of animal experiments, 48 kinds of single Chinese medicines with high tumor inhibition rate were screened, and 26 kinds of them were found to enhance phagocytosis by immune and cytokine level detection; or enhance cellular immunity: or enhance humoral immunity ; or increase the weight of thymus; or promote the proliferation of bone marrow cells; or enhance the function of T cells; or enhance the activity of LAK cells: or inhibit platelet coagulation and antithrombotics; or antiviral, anti-metastasis: or clear free radical base, etc.

The summary of anti-cancer mechanism of XZ-C immunomodulatory anti-cancer Chinese medication is:

(1) Activate the **body's immune cell system**, promote the enhancement of host defense mechanism effects, and restore the ability of immune response to cancer.

(2) Activate the immune cytokine system of the body's anti-cancer mechanism, enhance the host's immune defense mechanism, and improve the immune surveillance of immune cells in the body's blood circulation system.

(3) Protect **thymus, enhance immunity, protect marrow and generate blood, protect bone marrow physiological mechanism, stimulate bone marrow hematopoietic function, promote recovery of bone marrow function, increase white blood cell and red blood cell count, etc.**

(4) Reduce the adverse effects of radiotherapy and chemotherapy, and enhance the tolerance of the host.

(5) The progress of cancer is caused by the imbalance between the biological characteristics of cancer cells and the body's ability to suppress cancer. The immune regulation of XZ-C is to improve immunity and restore balance between the two.

(6) It can directly regulate the growth and differentiation of tumor cells and play a regulatory role in growth and differentiation.

(7) It can make the thymus gland enlarge and gain weight, so that the thymus no longer atrophy.

(8) Stimulate the host's anti-tumor immune response, enhance the body's anti-tumor ability, strengthen the sensitivity of cancer cells to the body's anti-cancer mechanism, and help kill cancer cells that are metastasizing.

XZ-C immune modulation Chinese medicine treatment of tumor can make the host produce a strong immune response to cancer cells, so as to achieve the purpose of treating cancer. XZ-C immunomodulatory anti-cancer Chinese medicine can cause the following immunological reactions in the host:

① *Enhance the regulation or restore the host's immune response to the tumor;*

② *Stimulate the body's inherent immune function and activate the host's immune defense system;*

③ *Restore immune function.*

As mentioned above, the mechanism of action of XZ-C immunomodulatory anti-cancer traditional Chinese medicine is basically similar to that of BRM, and clinical use also obtains the same therapeutic effect as BRM.

(4) Principles of cancer treatment

(Brief Introduction)

Cancer treatment should change the concept and establish a comprehensive treatment concept.

It is believed that cancer treatment should overcome the current one-sided treatment concept that only targets cancer cells, change the concept, and establish a comprehensive treatment concept.

In brief, it is proposed to establish a comprehensive treatment view that targets both the tumor and the host ; it is necessary to build a new therapy models so as to reach the better therapy results.

The goal of traditional therapies is simple, killing only cancer cells, but neglecting the host's own constraints on cancer cells. That means, the goal of the traditional cancer therapy is simply, only killing cancer cells, therefore ignores the host's own or inside ability to restrict the cancer cells

In order to obtain better treatment effects, it is necessary to establish a new treatment model.

After careful reflection, the author put forward the concept of "balance theory" that affects the occurrence and development of cancer.

If the goal of treatment is only to kill cancer cells, but only for one aspect, it is a one-sided view of treatment, and it is impossible to overcome cancer.

__The goal of treatment should be aimed at both the host and cancer cells, both killing the cancer cells and protecting the host, enhancing immune function, protecting Thymus and raising the immune function, protecting the bone marrow and producing blood, and enhancing the anti-cancer ability of the host.__

__This is the comprehensive treatment concept and it is possible to conquer cancer.__

How to establish a comprehensive view of cancer treatment?

A comprehensive view of cancer treatment, the goal is to target *__both the tumor and the host, from the two aspects of cancer cell biological characteristics and host body response, to study the clinical treatment plan of cancer:__*

(1) It is necessary to pay attention **to a set of anti-cancer systems inherent in the human body,** give full play to the role of its immune system, enhance immune surveillance, and prevent the escape of malignant cells.

(2) At the same time of radiotherapy and chemotherapy, the immune function of the host must also be improved.

Cancer cells cannot be killed solely by chemotherapeutics, but also by the body's anti-cancer ability, to eliminate cancer cells left by chemotherapy. It is because the cytotoxicity of chemotherapy has limited ability to kill cancer cells. That means that killing cancer cells cannot only depend on the chemotherapy, also depend on the host's ability to anticancer, in order to destroy the residual cancer cells.

① **The time of chemotherapy is limited and short.**

The effective time for chemotherapy to kill cancer cells in patients is only 1-5 days of intravenous infusion of drugs. It has the effect of killing cancer cells, and then it has no effect of killing cancer cells.

It is only a short time killing cancert (1-5 days), it can't be done once and for all.

After 5 days, the cancer cells continue to divide and proliferate.

After the chemotherapy is over, the efficacy will disappear, so it can only alleviate the improvement for a few weeks, and then the patient must rely on Anti-cancer ability of host immune function.

② **Chemotherapy is a "double-edged sword", which kills cancer cells and also kills the bone marrow hematopoietic cells of the host, and promotes the decline of immune function.**

Therefore, at the same time, chemotherapy must also protect, restore or enhance the host's immune function.

③ After the completion of radiotherapy and chemotherapy, the remaining cancer cells continue to divide, proliferate, and clone, and they still need to externally improve the host's anti-cancer ability to inhibit the development of tumors for a long time.

Since radiotherapy and chemotherapy both contribute to the decline in immune function, it is proposed that both radiotherapy and chemotherapy should be carried out simultaneously with immunotherapy, biological therapy, and XZ-C immunomodulatory anti-cancer traditional Chinese medicine treatment, and must be reformed into immuno+chemotherapy and immuno+radiotherapy.

(3) Improving the immune function of the host to inhibit tumor progression.

In the short term, cancer treatment relies on chemotherapeutic drugs to kill cancer cells, and in the long term, it depends on the immune function of the host and that immune surveillance eliminates the remaining cancer cells.

Therefore, a comprehensive treatment concept must improve the host's immune function through Thymus protection and increasing immune function to inhibit tumor progression.

Quoted from Chapter 5 of the original "Monograph"

(4) The principles of cancer treatment

(The detail explanation of Brief Introduction)

The principles of cancer treatment should change the concept and establish a comprehensive treatment concept

The main topics:

1. *It is to promote the establishment of a comprehensive treatment view for both tumor and host*
2. *How to establish a comprehensive view of cancer treatment?*
3. *Immune regulation and control are also the focus or main points of comprehensive cancer treatment*
4. *The goal of traditional therapy is simple, only kill cancer cells*
5. *Traditional therapy ignores the host's own restriction on cancer*

It is believed that the treatment of cancer should conquer the current one-sided treatment concept that only targets cancer cells, and should change the concept and **establish a comprehensive treatment concept**.

Because the process of cancer is the result of the mutual restriction of cancer cells and the function of the host body, the weakening of the host's anti-cancer power can lead to the **occurrence and development of tumors, and the enhancement of the host's anti-cancer power can control the development of cancer, just like "Seesaw", as one end goes up, the other goes down** or *just like "Rocker", this site rises and that site falls.*

Therefore, the treatment of cancer is not only to kill cancer cells, **but also to protect the host, not to harm the host, enhance the host's anti-cancer power, and establish a comprehensive view of cancer treatment.**

1. **It is recommended to establish a comprehensive treatment view for both the tumor and the host simultaneously or it is promoted to establish a comprehensive treatment view for both tumor and host:**

Since traditional therapies have not solved the problem in a real sense, it is necessary to establish a new treatment model to obtain better cancer treatment effects.

After careful thinking and analysis, the author puts forward the concept of *__"balance theory__"* that affects the occurrence and development of cancer:

a. Biological characteristics of cancer	b. Host's ability to restrict cancer

If Balance between the two is to maintain, the disease will be controlled	If Imbalance between the two is to happen, the disease progresses

Or the principles of "the balance theory" as the following:
The mode is as the following:

A. Host's ability to restrict it	<, =, >	B. Biological characteristics of cancer

The cancer recovers or be prevented when when A site is equal to or stronger than B sites (A site =/ > B site):

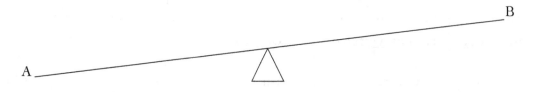

The cancer occurs when A site is weaker than B site(A site< B site):

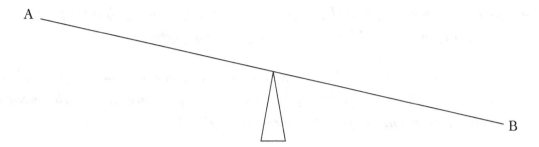

Therefore, the treatment target or goal must be aimed at both the tumor and the host:

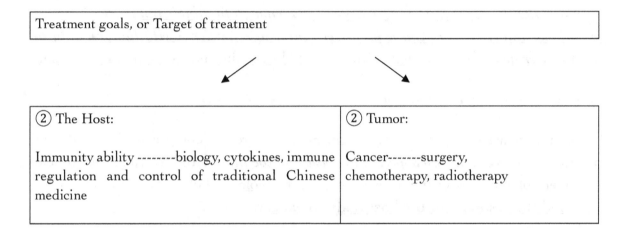

We believe that if the treatment target or target is only to kill cancer cells, it is only for one aspect, it is unilateral or one-sided. If the treatment target or target is also only immune regulation, it is also only for one aspect, and it is also unilateral or one-sided. With one-sided treatment, it is impossible to overcome cancer.

The treatment goal should be aimed at both the host and the cancer, both killing the cancer cells and protecting the host, enhancing immune function, protecting the Thymus and raising immune function, protecting the bone morrow and producing blood, and enhancing the host's ability to fight cancer.

This is the comprehensive treatment concept and it is possible to conquer cancer.

It was to follow up more than 3,000 patients who had undergone general and thoracic cancer surgery, and it was found that most patients relapsed and metastasized within 2-3 years after surgery.

After reviewing and reflecting on more than 50 years of experience and training in clinical oncology surgery, It is truly realized ***that in order to defeat cancer, it is*** *not only to kill cancer cells, but also to suppress tumors by improving the host's anti-cancer ability, which the specific treatment goals are as follows*:

(1) To control the occurrence and development of tumors, *the host should be considered first, and it should focus on how to suppress the occurrence and development of tumors by strengthening the anti-cancer ability of the host*.

(2) Strengthen the host's anti-cancer ability to inhibit tumor development and achieve tumor-bearing survival, thereby to prolong survival.

Try to make the host's anti-cancer force strong enough to inhibit tumor development for a long time, so as to achieve long-term survival of patients with tumors, only to treat cancer as a chronic disease. **Cancer is only considered as a chronic disease.**

2. *How to establish a comprehensive view of cancer treatment?*

The comprehensive view of cancer treatment and the goal of comprehensive treatment of cancer are to aim *at two aspects : the host and the tumor*, and to study the clinical treatment plan of cancer in terms of or from <u>the biological characteristics of cancer cells</u> **and the response of the host body to cancer.**

(1) It is necessary to pay attention **to a set of anti-cancer systems inherent in the human body, and give full play to the role of its immune system to enhance immune monitoring and prevent the escape of malignant cells.**

In fact, radiotherapy and chemotherapy can not kill cancer cells completely.

Due to the biological characteristics of cancer cells, the remaining cancer cells will continue to divide, proliferate, and clone, and they will multiply geometrically, leading to cancer recurrence and metastasis.

(2) At the same time as radiotherapy and chemotherapy, the immune function of the host must also be improved.

Killing cancer cells can not only rely on chemotherapy drugs, but also must rely on the body's anti-cancer ability to destroy the cancer cells left by chemotherapy.

It is because the cytotoxic drugs of chemotherapy have limited ability to kill cancer cells. The followings are the reasons why chemotherapy is limit:

① The time of chemotherapy is limited and short, and the chemotherapy drugs cannot be "once and forever", only it has the effect of killing cancer cells when intravenously administered as a chemotherapy drug.

After the completion of chemotherapy, the efficacy will disappear, even if it is done 4 or 6 times.

It only can manage or control for 2-3 months, and then must rely on the host's immune function to fight cancer.

② Chemotherapy is a "double-edged sword", which kills cancer cells and also kills the host's red marrow hematopoietic cells and immune cells, which promotes the decline of immune function.

Therefore, while it is to have chemotherapy, simultaneously it must also restore or enhance the host's immune function.

③ After the completion of radiotherapy and chemotherapy, the remaining tumor cells continue to divide, proliferate, and clone, and they still need to rely on improving the host's anti-cancer ability to inhibit tumor development for a long time.

Therefore, Dr. Xu Ze proposes that the current radiation therapy or chemotherapy should be carried out ***simultaneously with immunotherapy, biological therapy, XZ-C immunomodulatory anti-cancer traditional Chinese medicine treatment,*** **and must be reformed into immuno+chemotherapy and immuno+radiotherapy.**

(3) Improving the immune function of the host to inhibit tumor progression.

In the short term, cancer treatment relies on chemotherapeutic drugs to kill cancer cells, and in the long term, it depends on the host's immune function and immune surveillance to eliminate remaining cancer cells.

Therefore, a comprehensive treatment concept must improve the immune function of the host through Thymus protection and increasing immune function, in order to inhibit the progress of the tumor.

Cancer is a systemic disease.

It should study cancer and deliberate clinical treatment options from the biological characteristics and biological behavior of cancer.

The immune system is particularly suitable for removing a small amount of remaining cancer cells, especially Stationary phase (G0-G1) tumor cells or stem cells that are difficult to kill by radiotherapy or chemotherapy, which helps prolong the tumor-free survival of patients.

Radiotherapy and chemotherapy cannot kill all cancer cells, but only a part. The remaining cancer cells are destroyed by the host's immune cells.

Therefore, it is difficult to suppress cancer by relying solely on radiotherapy and chemotherapy.

Tumor immunotherapy is an important part of tumor biotherapy, and the important point or the focus of the comprehensive treatment concept.

The theoretical basis of tumor biotherapy is that Oldham founded the biological response regulation theory (ie, BRM theory) in 1982.

On this basis, it also proposed the **fourth modality of cancer treatment------- biotherapy** in 1984.

According to the BRM theory, under normal circumstances, the tumor and the body's defense are in a dynamic balance.

The occurrence, invasion and metastasis of the tumor are completely caused by the imbalance of the dynamic balance.

If the dysregulated state is adjusted to a normal level, the growth of the tumor can be controlled and resolved.

Biological therapy is to supplement, induce or activate **the biologically active cells (or) factors with cytotoxic activity inherent in the BRM system in vivo** to adjust the disordered state and control tumor growth.

Biological therapy is different from traditional therapy of surgery, radiotherapy and chemotherapy.

Biological tumor therapy mainly includes:

(1) adoptive infusion of live immune cells;

(2) Application of lymphokines/cytokines;

(3) Specific autoimmunity, including tumor vaccine and monoclonal antibody.

Under normal circumstances, the cells and humoral factors of the body's response system are under delicate or subtle control.

In the case of loss of balance, the body's reaction or response capacity will be significantly affected. The use of biological response modifiers is to restore the state of the body to a normal state to achieve the purpose of preventing and curing tumors.

The biological response modifier is to regulate the body's immune function and restore the suppressed body's immune system function. This type of medicine exerts its regulatory function by activating the body's immune system, and it comes from **microorganisms and plants mostly**.

3. *Immunomodulatory therapy is also the focus or main point of comprehensive cancer treatment*

XZ-C immunomodulatory anti-cancer Chinese medicine had been the experimental research for 4 years and the clinical verification for 26 years; XZ-C immunomodulatory anti-cancer Chinese medicine has been screened from natural medicine resources and has a BRM-like effect.

XZ-C immune-modulated anti-cancer Chinese medicine was selected from the experiment of 200 kinds of Chinese medicine by the author's laboratory. First, 200 kinds of Chinese medicine were screened one by one through the in vitro culture of cancer cells, and the direct damage of each Chinese medicine to the cancer cells in the culture tube was observed. The chemotherapeutic drug cyclophosphamide and normal cells cultured in test tubes were used as a control group for a comparative test of tumor inhibition rate. As a result, a batch of Chinese medications with a certain tumor suppressing rate on cancer cell proliferation was selected.

Then, it was to further manufacture tumor-bearing animal models, conduct in vivo anti-tumor rate screening experiments on tumor-bearing animal models for 200 kinds of traditional Chinese medicines one by one, and then analyze and evaluate after scientific, objective, and strict experimental screening. The experimental results prove that only 48 kinds of Chinese medicines do have a good tumor suppression rate.

Principles of application of XZ-C immunomodulatory Chinese medicine:

1. XZ-C immunomodulatory anti-cancer traditional Chinese medicine with BRM and BR1-like effects can enhance the body's immune response and strengthen the body's tumor immune surveillance.

2. When the cells are mutated or the tumor is very small, the effect is better.

Through surgery or radiation therapy, medical treatment works best or has the best effects when the tumor is minimized to the smallest sizes.

3. For those who have lost the chance of surgery, have poor health, and cannot tolerate radiotherapy or chemotherapy, immunotherapy has a certain effect, which can reduce the symptoms of patients and prolong the survival time of patients.

4. After radical tumor resection, in order to reduce recurrence and metastasis, XZ-C immunomodulatory anti-cancer Chinese medicine treatment is feasible.

After surgical removal of larger tumors, XZ-C immune regulation Chinese medicine treatment is also feasible to eliminate cancer cells that may remain and cancer cells that may spread in the distance.

5. If the tumor can not be removed, radiotherapy or chemotherapy can be used to kill the tumor cells in large quantities, so that the tumor load in the body is reduced and then treated with XZ-C immunomodulatory Chinese medicine.

In short, when the body's immune system is functional perfectly, the body can limit and eliminate tumors through its cellular and humoral immune responses. The growing tumor has many effects on the body's immune system, which can suppress the body's immune function and promote the development of the tumor.

Therefore, the cancer treatment plan must target both the host and the tumor. It is necessary to use theory to guide clinical practice, and at the same time to treat cancer cells and the anti-cancer ability of the host to establish a comprehensive treatment concept.

4. *The goal of traditional therapy is simple, just kill cancer cells*

Traditional cancer therapy believes that cancer is the continuous division and proliferation of cells, so cancer cells are the culprit.

The goal of cancer treatment must be to kill cancer cells. Both radiotherapy and chemotherapy only kill cancer cells.

Why did traditional therapies that only killed cancer cells not reduce mortality?

Why can't it prevent recurrence and metastasis?

Why can it only be relieved in the short term?

Why is it only relieved and not cured?

Is it really because the cancer can't be cured, or can it be cured by radiotherapy and chemotherapy alone?

What are the problems, defects and drawbacks of radiotherapy and chemotherapy itself, or is there a problem with the medical strategy of only killing cancer cells?

How many cancer cells did the patient kill every time it was hospitalized with chemotherapy?

How many cancer cells remain on the patient?

Is the drug used in this chemotherapy sensitive?

Is there drug resistance?

None of these can be known for sure. But it also suggests that traditional therapy does not meet the actual situation of the biological characteristics of cancer cells, it only considers the aspect of killing cancer cells, and ignores the role of host body functions.

5. *Traditional therapy ignores the host's own restriction on cancer*

In fact, the occurrence and development of tumors depends on the level of the host's immune function and the biological characteristics of the tumor itself, that is, the comparison between the biological characteristics of the tumor cells and the influence of the host on the restrictive factors.

If the two are balanced, they will be controlled. If these two is the imbalance, the cancer progresses.

For nearly half a century, all countries have been targeting cancer cell trials and seeking drugs to kill cancer cells. The idea is to be affected by the antibiotic-killing mode of bacteria and seek to kill cancer cells. As everyone knows, these are two completely different things. Antibiotics only kill bacteria but not normal cells, and can be used for drug sensitivity tests. The latter chemotherapeutic agent kills both cancer cells and normal cells, and is not yet able to be used for drug sensitivity tests.

Traditional therapy only focuses on killing cancer cells, but ignores the host's own anti-cancer system and the body's own anti-cancer ability, and ignores the host's anti-cancer cells (NK cell group, K cell group, LAK cell macrophage group, TK Cell population), anti-cancer factors (IFN, IL-1 TNF), ignore the role of tumor suppressor genes and tumor suppressor genes in the host (there are oncogenes and tumor suppressor genes in the human body, there are also cancer metastasis genes and Tumor suppressor metastasis gene), but also ignore the role of the host's neurohumoral system and endocrine hormones. These shadow factors have important adjustment, balance and stabilization effects on the host body, and should try to protect and activate various anti-cancer factors in the human body.

(5) Cancer treatment mode

(Brief Introduction)

Cancer treatment requires a scientifically designed treatment plan.

The occurrence of cancer is the loss of the balance between the body's immune anti-cancer ability and the development of the tumor. The loss of immune surveillance enables the tumor to develop further.

Treatment must restore the balance and stability between the host body and the tumor, or Treatment must restore the balance and stability of the two.

Cancer treatment requires a "multidisciplinary comprehensive treatment plan."

This program is an organic comprehensive treatment, which must be consistent with the actual condition of the patient's condition. In another word, **this plan is an organic comprehensive treatment and must be in line with the actual condition of the patient.**

The combination of multidisciplinary comprehensive treatment must have a reasonable theoretical basis and must be a comprehensive treatment view.

The new understanding of the host's impact or influence on tumor progression and metastasis *has important theoretical value and clinical guiding significance.*

When formulating anti-cancer invasion and anti-metastasis programs, it should be considered from both the tumor and host perspectives, and organically integrate or synthesize those *reasonable* disciplines, methods, technologies, and drugs with theoretical basis.

Based on the above analysis, **when formulating anti-cancer and anti-metastatic strategies in diagnosis, treatment, and drug development, *consideration should be given to both the tumor and the host.***

This may be a principle that fundamentally changes the current one-sided treatment plan that only kills cancer cells, and then establishes a comprehensive treatment concept.

How to combine multidisciplinary comprehensive treatment?

It is believed that, first of all, it should change the ideas, update the thinking, establish a comprehensive view of cancer treatment, and arrange interventions, adjustments, and treatment measures throughout the entire process of cancer occurrence, development, recurrence, and metastasis.

The current main treatment methods commonly used in various disciplines should conduct the comprehensive division of labor, and become organic coordination according to the full-course treatment and short-term treatment.

① Full-term treatment:

It is mainly by radical surgical treatment, the tumor has been removed, the lymph node has been removed, and then it is to carry out a long or full course of biological therapy, immunotherapy, cytokines, gene therapy, XZ-C immunomodulatory anti-cancer traditional Chinese medicine treatment, and Chinese and Western combined immunomodulatory traditional Chinese medicine treatment to enhance the host's anti-cancer immunity and regulate or control recurrence and metastasis.

It can be used for the entire process of cancer treatment.

② Short-term treatment.

It is mainly radiotherapy and chemotherapy, which can only be treated intermittently, or short-term assault to kill cancer cells, not the whole course or long-term treatment, nor can it be "once and forever", because it kills cancer cells during the 3-5 days of its use effect. After that, it has no effect on killing cancer cells. After short-term remission, the cancer cells continue to divide, proliferate, relapse, and metastasize, because they can only kill 4 or 6 cycles of cancer cells; after a long time, they may develop drug resistance.

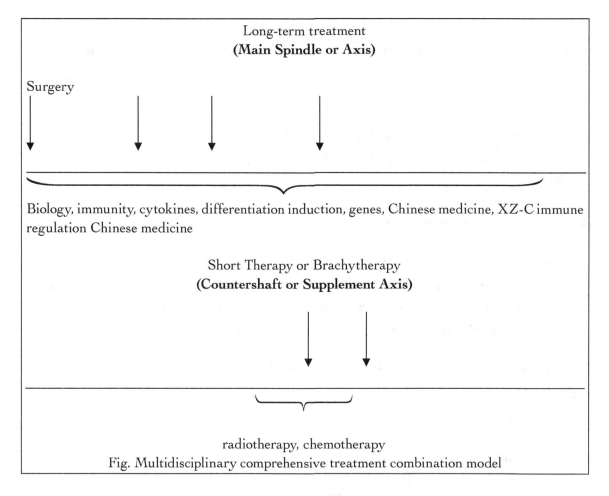

Fig. Multidisciplinary comprehensive treatment combination model

The above strategies of full-course treatment and short-course treatment are considered from the perspective of tumor and host, which may fundamentally change the current view of one-sided treatment that only kills cancer cells.

Short-term treatment only occupies a short-term stage in the entire course of cancer patients. Therefore, it should be adjuvant therapy (or vice axis), because it only targets unilateral cancer cells. It cannot become long range and excessive.

Traditional radiotherapy and chemotherapy are only for the factor of tumor, which is limited and one-sided, not comprehensive, so it is difficult to overcome cancer.

__Because the process of cancer is the result of an imbalance in regulation, it must address both the host and the tumor, and the host's response determines the final outcome. The cure should be through regulation and control rather than single killing.__

The full-term or full-course of treatment is the entire disease process from the occurrence, development, recurrence, metastasis and progression of cancer.

It is aimed at the two factors of tumor and host, and the tumor entity or tumor actual lesion is removed by radical surgery.

It is to treat the tumor through the biological treatment, immunotherapy, gene therapy, cytokine Treatment, XZ-C immunomodulatory Chinese medicine and other treatments, which is to improve the host's anti-cancer ability, and this scientific and organic comprehensive treatment is reasonable and scientific, consistent with the pathogenesis of cancer, pathophysiology, and biological characteristics of cancer cells and biological behavior, <u>therefore, it can conquer cancer.</u>

<u>Therefore, the full-term of treatment should be used as the main axis of cancer treatment, which is a radical cure or is the method for treating the root or essential of the disease.</u>

However, the short-term treatment should be used as a secondary treatment for cancer treatment, which **can only treat the symptoms** and can only be matched with the whole treatment, or which can only treat the symptoms and can only be used in conjunction with the entire treatment.

Quoted from Chapter 6 of the original "Monograph"

(5) Cancer treatment mode

(The extension of brief Introduction)

New combined model of multidisciplinary comprehensive treatment of cancer

1. Why is it to propose a new model of organic comprehensive treatment?

2. How to formulate a new model of multidisciplinary organic comprehensive treatment?

3. The initiatives for specific programs of multidisciplinary comprehensive treatment of cancer

It is believed that the combination of multidisciplinary comprehensive treatment must have a reasonable theoretical basis.

The new understanding that the host affects tumor progression and metastasis has important theoretical value and clinical guiding significance.

Before formulating anti-cancer and anti-metastatic strategies and comprehensive treatment plans, **it <u>should be reasonably consider the rationally based disciplines, methods, technologies, and drugs from the perspective of tumor and host, and integrate these organically.</u>**

<u>**This just is the comprehensive treatment concept**</u>.

In the 21ˢᵗ century, cancer treatment has entered the era of multidisciplinary comprehensive treatment.

<u>***The current status of comprehensive treatment***</u> is that the three traditional treatment methods are the main body, and how to apply other comprehensive treatment methods is mostly determined by the first clinic department.

Most patients are first diagnosed as chemotherapy department, so chemotherapy is first followed by radiotherapy. If the patient is a radiotherapy department for the first time, radiotherapy is first given and followed by chemotherapy. If the first diagnosis is surgery and there are indications for surgery, surgery is performed first, followed by chemotherapy or radiotherapy. If there is no indication for surgery, radiotherapy and chemotherapy are given.

As a result of such comprehensive treatment, many patients still have relapses and metastases, and even some patients suffer from immune failure.

However, biological therapy, immunotherapy, induced differentiation therapy, cytokine therapy, and combined Chinese and Western medicine immunomodulation therapy have not yet been included in most oncologists' treatment plans.

1. Why should it be proposed the new model of organic comprehensive treatment?

Cancer therapy research must be based on tumor biology, and the two must coincide. In other words, the research of cancer therapy must be based on tumor biology, and the two must be consistent.

Tumor biology has developed to the level of molecular biology, cytokines, and genes, but the current theoretical basis of traditional cancer therapy is still at the cellular level half a century ago.

In the past 60 years, the research trend and clinical application status of antitumor drugs at home and abroad have shown that traditional anti-neoplastic drugs are subject to more and more restrictions due to large adverse reactions, poor targeting, and the tumor's resistance to drugs.

It can be considered that the research of anticancer drugs has reached a new stage, and it will face the renewal of theory, technology and thinking.

Traditional therapies, traditional ideas and working methods based on the theory that cytotoxic drugs kill cancer cells are being impacted.

Since the 1980s, medical molecular science, molecular immunology, immunopharmacology, traditional Chinese medicine immunopharmacology, and cytokine science have developed rapidly, and new biotherapeutics have emerged to promote the development of cancer therapeutics.

Biotherapy, immunotherapy, differentiation inducers, biological response modifiers, molecular-level Chinese and Western medicine combined with immunomodulatory Chinese medicine are gradually on the stage.

The development of new tumor vaccines and gene therapy in recent years has provided attractive prospects for cancer treatment.

It is believed that cancer treatment requires a scientifically designed treatment plan. The occurrence of cancer is a loss of balance between the body's immune anti-cancer ability and tumor development. It loses immune surveillance and further development of the tumor. Treatment must make both restore balance and stability.

2. How to formulate a multi-disciplinary organic comprehensive treatment plan?

(1) The treatment of cancer requires a "multidisciplinary organic comprehensive treatment plan".

This plan is organic comprehensive treatment, which must be in accordance with or conform the actual condition of the patient's condition:

① **The biological characteristics of cancer cells are that after malignant cells in the body become cancer cells, they continue to divide, proliferate, clone, and throughout the entire process of cancer occurrence, development, metastasis, and recurrence.**

Therefore, the treatment measures must also implement the corresponding control and treatment in the whole process, rather than focusing only on a certain stage of the disease process.

② **Cancer is a development process.** Cancer cells are characterized by uncontrolled infinite reproduction, and their malignant transformation process is the result of unbalanced regulation and control.

There is a certain response relationship between the tumor and the host, **and the host's response determines the final result. In other words, a** certain response relationship is maintained between the tumor and the host, and the response of the host determines the final result.

③ According to the biological behavior of cancer cells, the multiple steps and muti-links of cancer cell metastasis, the eight steps, three stages and two points and one line of cancer cell metastasis, intervene and block cancer cells that are in the process of metastasis, it adopts or takes a new model of scientific organic combination comprehensive treatment.

(2) **The combination of multidisciplinary comprehensive treatment must have a reasonable theoretical basis, and it must be a comprehensive treatment concept, and the new understanding that the host affects tumor progression and metastasis has important theoretical value and clinical guiding significance.**

When formulating anti-cancer invasion and anti-metastasis programs, it should be considered from the perspective of tumor and host, and organically synthesize the reasonable and theoretical based disciplines, methods, technologies, and drugs.

What are the main determinants in the occurrence, development and metastasis of cancer?

Is it a host or a tumor?

Is it the immune and anti-cancer ability of the host organism, or the invasion and metastatic power of cancer cells?

Over the past half century, research has focused on cancer cells themselves, and countries are targeting how to kill cancer cells.

Therefore, although traditional treatments that only kill cancer cells have made some striking progress, they have not fundamentally solved the problem. They are just a cure for the symptoms without curing the essential.

In recent years, people have turned more attention to host factors, through the experimental research on the etiology, pathogenesis, pathophysiology of cancer and the mechanism of cancer invasion and metastasis, it is to explore the interaction between the host's anti-cancer immune function and tumor, and find the regulatory mechanism of cancer cell invasion and metastasis.

Therefore, it is to proposes the concept of "balance", that is, cancer is caused by the loss of balance between the biological characteristics of cancer cells and the host's immune function. If the balance is restored, the cancer will be controlled, and the treatment must be aimed at both the host and the tumor to restore balance and stability.

By the experimental explore of the interaction and relationship between this host and tumor and the analysis of clinical practice experience and lessons, whether is it cancer cells or host factors that determine the occurrence, development, metastasis and recurrence of cancer? *What is the cause of cancer death? Why does cancer cause death?*

It has realized that the main cause of death of cancer patients is <u>metastasis and relapse</u>, but how does relapse and metastasis cause death?

Our preliminary analysis, thinking, and experience are that the cancer patients died of complications and immune function failure, leading to this final result, which should be considered as two factors : **the tumor itself and host factors.**

The disease process of the cancer development can simply be described as the following:

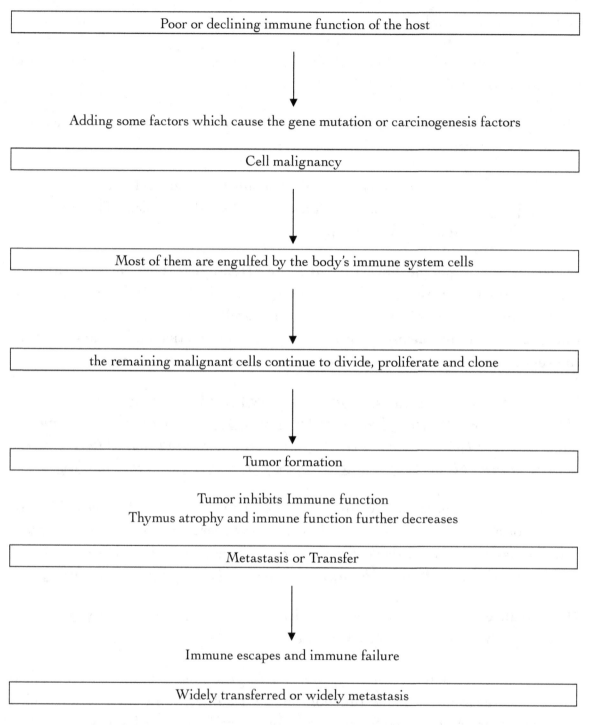

Poor or declining immune function of the host

Adding some factors which cause the gene mutation or carcinogenesis factors

Cell malignancy

Most of them are engulfed by the body's immune system cells

the remaining malignant cells continue to divide, proliferate and clone

Tumor formation

Tumor inhibits Immune function
Thymus atrophy and immune function further decreases

Metastasis or Transfer

Immune escapes and immune failure

Widely transferred or widely metastasis

__It is believed that it is the interaction between cancer cells and the host microenvironment and immune anti-cancer ability that ultimately determine the progress of cancer, whether and when metastases form.__

The disclosure of this interaction regulation mechanism has important theoretical value and clinical guiding significance, and in the aspect of formulating anti-cancer and anti-metastatic strategies and the development of new drugs, it should be considered from **two perspectives of tumor factors and host factors,** which provide a theoretical basis for us to find effective methods and develop new drugs for prevention and treatment.

The XZ-C anti-cancer traditional Chinese medications researched and developed by us are the theoretical basis and experimental basis for Thymus protection and increasing immune function, bone marrow protection and promotion of blood production studied and developed from the enhancement of host factors.

Based on the above analysis, the diagnosis, treatment, drug development, and anti-cancer and anti-metastatic strategies should be considered from two aspects or two angles, that is, the tumor and the host, or from the perspective of tumor and host.

This may be a principle which should be followed for which it fundamentally changes the current one-sided treatment plan that only kills cancer cells, and then it establishes a comprehensive view of treatment, or a comprehensive treatment concept.

3. The proposal of specific plans for multidisciplinary comprehensive treatment of cancer

How to combine multidisciplinary comprehensive treatment?

It is believed that first of all, it should change the concepts and update the thinking, establish a comprehensive view of cancer treatment, and arrange measures or strategies of interventions, adjustments, and treatments throughout the entire process of cancer occurrence, development, recurrence, and metastasis.

According to the main treatment methods commonly used in various disciplines, according to full term treatment or short term treatment, it is to give the comprehensive division of labor and organic cooperation, which are as the following(Fig. below):

(1) Full-term treatment.

Radical surgical treatment is the main method. The tumor has been removed and the lymph nodes have been removed.

Then long-term or full course of biological therapy, immunotherapy, cytokine therapy, differentiation induction therapy, gene therapy, combined Chinese and Western immunotherapy, XZ-C immunomodulated anti-cancer traditional Chinese medicine treatment can be conducted, to enhance the host's anti-cancer immunity, regulate and control the recurrence and metastasis.

They can be used in the entire process of cancer disease treatment.

(2) Short-term treatment:

It is mainly radiotherapy and chemotherapy, which is staged treatment or intermittent treatment, or short-term assault treatment to kill cancer cells.

It is not a full-course or long-term treatment, nor can it be "once and for all."

It is because it can only kill cancer cells for 4 cycles or 6 cycle, and over time, it may be resistant to medication.

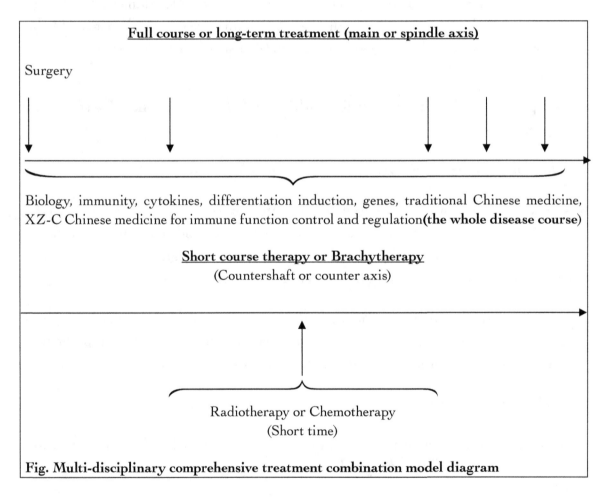

Full course or long-term treatment (main or spindle axis)

Surgery

Biology, immunity, cytokines, differentiation induction, genes, traditional Chinese medicine, XZ-C Chinese medicine for immune function control and regulation**(the whole disease course)**

Short course therapy or Brachytherapy
(Countershaft or counter axis)

Radiotherapy or Chemotherapy
(Short time)

Fig. Multi-disciplinary comprehensive treatment combination model diagram

The above strategies for full-course treatment and short-course treatment are considered from the perspective of **tumor factors and host**s, which may fundamentally change the current one-sided treatment view that only kills cancer cells.

Short-term treatment only occupies a short-term stage in the entire course of cancer patients, so it should be adjuvant therapy (or called a secondary axis), because it only targets unilateral cancer cells.

① **Biological characteristics of cancer cells:**

The formation of cancer originates from the malignant transformation of a single cell, the cancer cells continue to divide and proliferate,

Cancer is a developmental or progressive process, not a form or shape, or solid or entity(cancer is continuing changing over the time).

Therefore, every effort of killing cancer is made to treat cancer cells is impossible to kill cancer cells totally or completely.

As long as cancer cells remain, they will continue and persist to divide, proliferate, and relapse. Moreover, chemotherapy cannot kill tumor stem cells. Cancer stem cells must continue to divide and proliferate, forming cancer cells. **Therefore, the treatment method that only kills cancer cells does not conform to the biological characteristics and biological behavior of cancer cells.**

② **The effective time of cytotoxic killing is time-limited.**

It is only effective when the drug is used. After the time, it is invalid, and it cannot be "one time forever."

Its action time is limited. The remaining 10^6-10^7 cancer cells will eventually be destroyed by the host's immunity, not to mention that cancer stem cells continue to form cancer cells, so radiotherapy and chemotherapy can only relieve for several months and cannot be cured.

③ Chemotherapy is only a first-order kinetics to kill cancer cells, and its lethality is limited. It can only kill 10^6-10^7 cancer cells.

④ The chemotherapy drug is a "double-edged sword", which not only kills cancer cells but also kills normal cells, bone marrow hematopoietic cells and immune cells of the host, resulting in a decline in the host's immune function.

Traditional radiotherapy and chemotherapy are only targeted at cancer cell tumors. They are limited, one-sided, and not comprehensive, making it difficult to

overcome cancer. Because the process of canceration is the result of an imbalance in regulation and control, both the host and tumor must be targeted, and the *host's response determines the final result.* The cure should be through regulation and control rather than only or single killing.

(3) The full treatment is the treatment from the entire disease process of the occurrence, development, recurrence, metastasis and progression of cancer and is the treatment which is directed at the two factors of tumor and host and is that radical surgery is used to remove the entity of the cancer focus, and the treatment for using biotherapy, immunotherapy, gene therapy cytokines, and immunomodulatory Chinese medicine to improve the host's anti-cancer ability.

This scientific and organic view of comprehensive treatment is reasonable and scientific. It is consistent with the pathogenesis and pathophysiology of cancer, and with the biological characteristics and biological behavior of cancer cells, so it is also possible to conquer cancer.

Therefore, full-course treatment should be the mainstay of cancer treatment, with surgical treatment as the mainstay. At the same time, biotherapy, immunomodulatory therapy, cytokine therapy, gene therapy, differentiation induction therapy, traditional Chinese medicine immunomodulatory therapy, etc. are used throughout the entire process of cancer therapy. This is the cure for the root cause. The short-term treatment should be the secondary axis of cancer treatment, mainly radiotherapy and chemotherapy, and cooperate with the whole course of treatment.

The author believes that the above new model of combined multidisciplinary comprehensive treatment has reasonable theoretical guidance and is in line with the actual condition of the patient's condition. It is reasonable and scientific.

After half a century of experience and lessons from clinical case treatment practice, it has been proven that a single cancer cell killer cannot control the cancer and cannot defeat it. It is a one-sided treatment and is not comprehensive.

The goal or target of cancer treatment should be to both the host and the tumor. Which side is the main one and who decides the ultimate fate of the cancer patient should also be a factor of both the tumor and the host.

It must update our thinking, change our concepts, and establish a comprehensive view of cancer treatment in the entire process of cancer occurrence, development, recurrence, and metastasis.

A new treatment model of "main axis + counter axis or secondary axis" should be established, which will be a reasonable and scientific design, which has both theoretical basis and guidance and is _in line with the actual condition of the disease._

<u>People-oriented</u> must be used to eliminate the adverse effects of radiotherapy and chemotherapy as much as possible **to improve the safety of patients**. Every drug and every technology must have an accurate understanding of its toxicity and safety to ensure a reasonable theoretical basis to guide clinical practice.

In short, the treatment of cancer, whether it is early, middle, or late, requires comprehensive multidisciplinary treatment. There must be reasonable theory to guide clinical practice.

<u>In the past 20 years, there have been many reports on the treatment of cancer by traditional Chinese medicine, and its prospects have attracted people's attention</u>. Especially with the continuous deepening of medical and immunological research, people have recognized that the disorder of the body's immune system is closely related to the occurrence and development of tumors.

Traditional Chinese medicine has unique characteristics and advantages in treating tumors by adjusting the body's immune function.

The immunomodulatory effects of traditional Chinese medicine and the development of traditional Chinese medicine immunomodulatory drugs will be valued and favored worldwide.

The combination of XZ-C immunomodulatory Chinese medicine and surgery, radiotherapy, and chemotherapy can give full play to its immune regulation in the treatment process, significantly prolong the patient's survival period, improve the patient's quality of life, and reflect the characteristics and advantages of traditional Chinese medicine in treating cancer, **but The weakness is that the changes to the tumor itself are not very significant**.

Due to the various mechanisms and effects of the above-mentioned methods on cancer treatment, their efficacy is also different, and each has its own weaknesses.

This requires to measure the advantages and disadvantages of various therapies, and the gains and losses for patients.

What are the advantages and disadvantages of using this therapy, what will the patient gain and lose?

Each of these therapies should take their own strengths and complement each other's shortcomings, and organically and reasonably combine these ***therapies to form a comprehensive treatment plan for cancer,*** so that the adverse reactions of drugs can be significantly reduced, the quality of life of patients can be improved, and the overall survival time of the patients can be extended.

Over the past 16 years, the author has practiced comprehensive treatment of more than 12,000 patients with advanced cancer using surgery + XZ-C immunomodulatory anti-cancer traditional Chinese medicine, etc.

As a result, most of them have obtained improved quality of life, stable lesions, controlled metastasis, and the patient survival with tumor, and significantly prolonging life.

(6)   The principles of cancer metastasis treatment

(Brief introduction explanation)

1. ***The key to win or tackle main issues of cancer or cancer research is to resist metastasis or anti-metastasis***
2. ***The basic principle of cancer treatment is anti-metastasis***
3. ***The main feature of the new concept of cancer treatment, that is, or namely control of metastasis***

It can be seen from clinical medical practice in the past 100 years that the three traditional therapies: surgery, radiotherapy, and chemotherapy have achieved good results in the treatment of malignant tumors.

Many patients have undergone radiotherapy and chemotherapy, their tumors have shrunk significantly, but the tumors recurred, enlarged, and metastasized soon afterwards.

Although radiotherapy or chemotherapy can be performed again, most of them have very poor results and eventually die of cancer metastasis and recurrence.

Dr. Xu Ze summarized the positive and negative experience and lessons of clinical practice cases over the past 60 years, combined with long-term experimental research and clinical practice experience, and gained the following new understandings, proposed new theoretical concepts, and advocated the implementation of new treatment strategies.

1. The key to win or tackle main issues of cancer or cancer research is to resist metastasis or anti-metastasis

Metastasis is the main cause of cancer death, so metastasis is the key to cancer treatment.

Since the 20th century, the goal of cancer treatment has been to kill cancer cells against primary and metastatic tumors.

Although after a century of hard work, the fatality rate of cancer still ranks first among human diseases.

The main reason for such a high mortality rate is metastasis.

The original traditional therapy failed to reduce the long-term high mortality rate. The main reason for its failure was the failure to target metastasis and control the transfer.

Today, the most important problem in cancer treatment is how to resist metastasis.

If the problem of cancer metastasis cannot be solved, cancer treatment cannot leap forward.

Therefore, one of the goals of 21 cancer treatment should be anti-metastasis.

Recognizing the above problems prompts us to update our thinking, change our concepts, and find new ways to fight against metastasis and overcome cancer.

For this reason, it is proposed that, according to the biological characteristics of cancer and the biological behavior of cancer metastasis, to analyze and understand the host immune status, the multi-step and multi-link process of cancer metastasis, and molecular transfer mechanism, etc., it is to propose a new treatment model for anti-cancer metastasis.

Academician Tang Zhaoxian in Liver Cancer Research Institute of Fudan University put forward: **"If you don't study cancer metastasis, it will be empty talk to improve the efficacy."** on November 9, 2007, in the article "Clinical Research on Cancer Metastasis".

The international community has attached great importance to the research of tumor metastasis since the 1990s, and established the International Metastasis Research Society (Metastasis Research Society), and published the journal "Clinical and Experimental Metastasis"; the Cancer Metastasis Research Association has also been established in Tokyo, Japan.

The study of domestic transfer started late. In 1996, Professor Gao Jin published **"Invasion and Metastasis of Cancer---Basic Research and Clinic"**, the first monograph on cancer metastasis in China.

In 2003, Academician Tang Zhaota's monograph **"The basis and clinical practice of liver cancer metastasis and recurrence"** was published.

It is to put forward in the monograph: *"**The next important goal of primary liver cancer research----------the prevention and treatment of recurrence and metastasis**"*, *"**Metastasis and recurrence have become a bottleneck to further improve the survival rate of liver cancer, and are also one of the most important difficulties in overcoming cancer.**"* These academic monographs have promoted domestic scholars' attention to the research of tumor metastasis.

In 2006, Professor Xu Ze published the book "New Concepts and New Methods of Cancer Metastasis Treatment" and put forward some related theories.

2. The basic principle of cancer treatment is anti-metastasis

(1) Targeting the biological behavior of cancer cells, that is, or namely the unique behavior of <u>invasion and metastasis or transfer.</u>

Metastasis is malignant behavior.

It is well known that the fundamental difference between benign tumors and malignant tumors is that the former does not metastasize while the latter metastasizes.

If there are ways to prevent cancer cells from metastasis, then malignant tumors may become benign tumors.

85%-95% of cancer deaths are caused by metastasis.

If metastasis does not occur, most patients will not die. If it does not metastasize or control metastasis, cancer will become less scary.

Therefore, the principle of cancer treatment should be the formulation of anti-metastatic treatment plans and intervention plans, the development of anti-metastatic drugs, and the design of encirclement and interception of cancer cells during metastasis, cutting off or blocking one or several links during metastasis with the multi-step, multi-link, multi-factor, and multi-gene to achieve control of transfer or metastasis.

(2) How to resist metastasis or how to conduct anti-cancer?

The biological characteristics and biological behavior of cancer cells are invasion and metastasis.

The reason why cancer is malignant is mainly because its invasion and metastasis can cause widespread harm to the human body.

For more than a century, the three traditional treatments have targeted primary cancer masses and metastatic cancer masses. Surgical removal of primary cancer masses or radiotherapy and other local treatments have been used to treat metastatic cancer masses. It is generally believed that the primary cancer mass and metastatic cancer mass are visible or tangible, which is a local problem and can be treated by means of surgery or radiotherapy.

Looking back and reflecting on the author's 50 years of clinical practice, based on the above knowledge, many "radical cures" of various cancers of the chest and abdomen have been performed. However, in 1985, the author followed up 3000 patients after surgery, and **suddenly realized that how to prevent postoperative recurrence and metastasis is the core issue that determines the long-term effect of cancer.**

The primary tumor mass or metastasis may be a local manifestation, <u>while distant metastasis is a systemic problem</u>.

Since the 1970s, in view of the high recurrence and metastasis rate of cancer after surgery, a series of adjuvant chemotherapy after surgery has been used to control recurrence after surgery, and chemotherapy has even been started before surgery (such as breast cancer), but the results are not satisfactory.

In many patients, postoperative adjuvant chemotherapy has failed to prevent recurrence and metastasis. ***In some cases, intensive chemotherapy has promoted immune failure.***

These are things that clinicians should seriously and calmly think, review, analyze, and reflect on. ***<u>The focus of cancer treatment should also shift to how to prevent recurrence and resist metastasis.</u>***

In the past 20 years, great progress has been made in the understanding of the molecular mechanism of cancer metastasis. So far, there are still no good methods at home and abroad for anti-cancer metastasis.

Although many new anticancer drugs have appeared in recent years, the efficacy has not been improved satisfactorily. *Some of the reasons why surgery for advanced cancers cannot be radically removed are distant lymph node metastases.*

<u>Therefore, inhibiting cancer metastasis is the key to reducing cancer mortality and improving curative effect</u>.

The goal of traditional therapies is relatively simple, only killing cancer cells, which is not entirely consistent with the current known actual conditions of cancer biological characteristics, such as the invasion behavior of cancer cells, metastasis links and multiple steps, the molecular biological mechanism of metastasis, the body's immune reactivity and the inducement of recurrence, etc.

At present, people have realized that anti-cancer drugs may not necessarily prevent metastasis, and anti-metastatic drugs may not necessarily kill cancer cells.

Therefore, it is believed that the key to current cancer research is anti-metastasis, and research on anti-metastasis is the core topic of cancer treatment.

3. *The main feature of the new concept of cancer treatment, that is, namely control of metastasis*

Killing cancer cells in the human body should rely on two forces:

<u>One is the external forces of surgery, radiotherapy, and chemotherapy;</u>

<u>The second is the internal strength of the patient's own immune function</u>.

Drugs, surgery, and various treatment techniques are certainly important for the treatment of patients, *but the body's own immune function is even more important.*

Many problems must be solved by the patient's own strength, such as nutritional problems. Even if a sufficient amount of nutrition is given, if the patient's body cannot absorb and utilize it, it will be difficult to achieve the goal.

Another example is the wound healing problem, which must rely on the patient's own healing function, and external factors can only affect or promote its healing.

The body's own immune function can kill cancer cells.

Documents indicate that a very small tumor (1-8g) can release millions or tens of millions of cancer cells into the bloodstream within 24 hours, but the human immune system can remove most of cancer cell in the blood (99.9%). And less than 0.1% of cancer cells survive and continue to grow into metastatic cancer.

The author's experimental data show that Kunming mice were injected with $10^5 S_{180}$ malignant cells in the tail vein. After 24 hours, the mice could eliminate 99% of the cancer cells by relying on their own immune function.

Oral administration of $XZ\text{-}C_1$ and $XZ\text{-}C_4$ immunomodulatory Chinese medicines to mice can eliminate more cancer cells.

In the past 10 years, according to the clinical data of the Anti-cancer Metastasis Laboratory of Wuhan Shuguang Oncology Specialty Clinic, the routine use of $XZ\text{-}C_1$ and $XZ\text{-}C_4$ on patients can indeed eliminate a certain amount of cancer cells on the way to metastasis.

The human body has certain anti-cancer ability. This is because the human body has a complete anti-cancer system such as:

1, anti-cancer effects against cancer cell populations (NK cell population, K cell population, LAK cell population, macrophage cell population, TK cell population),

2, anti-cancer effect of anti-cancer factor system (IFN, IL-2, TNF, LT),

3, the role of tumor suppressor genes and tumor suppressor metastasis genes,

4, the role of neurohumoral and endocrine hormones.

These anti-cancer systems in the human body and their effects play a role in regulating, balancing and stabilizing the body's anti-cancer functions. Therefore, they must be protected, activated and mobilized.

The occurrence, development and metastasis of cancer are closely related to the decline of the body's immune function.

Cancer can directly invade immune organs and cause immune function decline or suppression. It can also release immunosuppressive factors to reduce host immunity or induce an increase in suppressive cells in the body.

When cancer occurs, the host thymus has been suppressed, and chemotherapy will suppress the bone marrow, as if "frost addes on snow, or the worse causes the worse."

Traditional treatment methods ignore the human body's own anti-cancer ability, and ignore the anti-cancer powers of the host, such as anti-cancer cells, anti-cancer factors, and anti-metastasis genes, which damage the entire central immune organs without effective protection.

This is the reason why the efficacy of traditional therapies cannot be improved.

It is believed that in cancer treatment, attention must be paid to exerting and relying on the power of the host's own anti-cancer system.

The main feature of the new concept of cancer treatment is to control metastasis and protect patient immune function, rather than simply killing cancer cells.

(7)　The new concept of cancer metastasis treatment

(The description of Brief Introduction)
Targeting or aiming cancer cell population on the way

The main topic :
The main manifestations of cancer existing in the human body

1. *The new concept of cancer treatment believes that there are three forms*
2. *The goal of cancer treatment should be for the above three existing forms*
3. *The process of research and understanding of the third form of cancer in the human body*
4. *Traditional cancer therapy believes that there are two forms*

It is carefully analyzed, summarized, summarized about 60 years of clinical treatment experience in tumor surgery and more than 30 years of laboratory research results, then it is to form a unique new understanding and new concept of cancer metastasis, and it is to propose the new technologies and new methods for cancer anti-metastasis therapy.

Its main contents include:

① Three manifestations or existing forms of cancer in the human body;

② The "two points and one line" theory of the whole process of cancer development;

③ The "eight steps and three stages" theory of cancer metastasis;

④ The second field or area of human anti-cancer metastasis therapy;

⑤ The "three steps" of cancer metastasis treatment;

⑥ A series of XZ-C immune regulation and control anti-cancer Chinese medicine preparations independently researched and developed.

The following new understandings, new theories, and new concepts have not been mentioned in the literature and textbooks so far. They are all the experience and lessons of the author after half a century of clinical practice and more than 30 years of experimental research, analysis, reflection, and insight into theories.

These theoretical innovations have also become the author's unique theoretical system for the new concept of anti- cancer metastatic therapy, with independent intellectual property rights of independent innovation and original innovation.

1. The new concept of cancer treatment thinks that there are three forms

A new theoretical understanding is first published at the international conference, that is, the third form of cancer in the human body is cancer cells that are on the way to metastasis.

The new concept of cancer metastasis treatment believes that there are three manifestations of cancer in the human body:

The first type is primary cancer;
The second type is metastatic cancer;
The third type is a group of cancer cells on the way to metastasis.

It is just these cancer cell populations on the way of metastasis that may be the main reason for recurrence and metastasis after cancer surgery.

Cancer cells that are on the way to metastasis are invisible to the naked eye during surgery.

For example, during "radical gastric cancer surgery", gastric cancer masses and metastatic enlarged lymph nodes can be seen.

However, it is not possible to see whether there are cancer cells in the bloodstream of the gastric wall vein and the hepatic portal vein, and how many cancer cells there are.

Where did these cancer cells in the venous bloodstream have reached?

Whether these clusters of cancer cells that were squeezed into the venous blood stream by the touch during the operation have reached the gastric vein?

Or has it reached the hepatic portal vein or even the branch of the intrahepatic portal vein?

During surgical exploration and removal of gastric cancer masses and lymph node dissection, it is impossible not to touch the cancer masses, because the operation of the hands will inevitably cause a large number of cancer cells to be squeezed off and flow into the blood circulation through the tumor veins. It rushes into the blood stream of the portal vein, but the surgeon cannot see it.

These cancer cells drifting into the bloodstream of the portal vein of the liver flow to the portal vein system of the liver.

Normally, various immune cells in the portal vein will carry out immune surveillance of cancer cells entering the blood circulation of the portal vein of the liver and carry out phagocytosis processing.

However, in a short period of time, the immune cells of the portal venous system cannot deal with these sudden influx of cancer cells.

After some time, some cancer cells escaped immune surveillance; cancer cells that survive through the impact of blood flow may implant in the liver sinusoids, generate blood vessels and form intrahepatic metastases.

This is a phenomenon and a fact, but it was never thought of or discovered in the past. It is a dynamic form of cancer cells in the human body.

In our Research Laboratory of Anti-cancer Metastasis and Recurrence, Institute of Experimental Surgery, through the analysis and research of more than 10,000 outpatient cancer patients metastasis, **it is found that the essence of metastasis is cancer cells in the process of metastasis or the cancer cells on the way of metastasis.**

The target of anti-metastasis and the "target" of treatment should be targeted at cancer cells on the way to metastasis, which is the third form of cancer in the human body.

Since this point was not recognized in the past, it was only targeted at the primary and metastatic cancer foci and tried to treat it and to shrink or eliminate it.

Who knows that shrinking a lump does not mean that it will not metastasize. The long-term effects of traditional therapies often fail due to recurrence and metastasis. This shows that the lack of understanding of traditional therapy has led to the failure of its long-term efficacy.

2. The goal of cancer treatment should be for the above three-existing forms

The goal or "target" of cancer treatment should be for the three forms of cancer that exist in the human body, namely, one of the goals of treatment, for the primary lesion; the second goal of treatment, for the metastatic cancer; *the third goal of treatment is to target the cancer cell population on the way to metastasis.*

(I) Targeting cancer cells on the way to metastasis is the key to winning cancer metastasis

***It is proposed that the third manifestation of cancer in the human body is the metastasis of cancer cells, cancer cell populations and micro-cancer thrombi in the multi-step and multi-factor process of metastasis or** that are in the process of metastasis with multiple steps and multiple factors.* It is because this problem has not been recognized by people so far, nor has it attracted enough attention, even more there is no specific discussion on how to diagnose and treat methods and countermeasures.

In fact, the key to anti-cancer metastasis is to encircle, block or interfere with cancer cells in the process of metastasis, and to cut off the new treatment model. In other words, in fact, the new treatment model of encircling, blocking or interfering with cancer cells on the way to metastasis, cutting off the metastasis pathway is the key to win cancer metastasis.

(2) Targeting cancer cells on the way to metastasis may cause changes and updates in tumor diagnosis and treatment

This new theory or new theoretical understanding, which argumentation has already been confirmed, may lead to a series of changes and updates of chain reaction-like tumor **diagnosis and treatment**, such as:

1, changes and updates in the understanding of the concept of cancer treatment;
2, changes and updates in the understanding of the goals or "targets" of cancer treatment;
3, changes and updates in cancer diagnosis methods;
4, it can cause major changes and updates on the research and development of new anti-cancer and anti-metastatic drugs.
5, it can lead major changes and updates in cancer treatment models and treatment methods.
6, it can lead the change and update for the research on cancer metastasis and recurrence from the cell-level oncology of cytopathological morphology to molecular biology and gene expression on the molecular level.

(3) Targeting cancer cells on the way to metastasis will bring new hope to the beating against cancer

(1) The new concept of cancer awareness proposed by the author believes that there are three manifestations:

The first manifestation is the primary cancer;
The second manifestation is metastatic cancer;

The third manifestation is the metastasis of cancer cells, cancer cell populations, and <u>microcancer thrombi on the way to metastasis</u>.

This new concept is relatively complete and comprehensive. It clarifies the dynamic relationship, causality and subordination between the three. It is a complete new concept of cancer therapy, which comprehensively explains the whole process of cancer development and how to control the whole process of cancer metastasis.

The proposal of this new doctrine has brought new hope for beating against cancer.

(2) Traditional cancer treatment methods believe that there are two manifestations:

the first manifestation is the primary cancer;
the second manifestation is the metastatic cancer.

This traditional therapeutic concept has been used for more than 100 years, and its therapeutic goals or "targets" are for these two manifestations-----primary cancer or metastatic cancer.

Treating these two "targets" in isolation, the dynamic relationship, causality, and subordination between the two are not considered, such as **how the primary cancer foci formed into metastatic cancer foci**, and how **to prevent or to stop** its metastasis, tec.

Therefore, the traditional concept of cancer therapy is incomplete, imperfect, and flawed or defective, because it ignores the cancer cells in the process of metastasis, and metastasis is the most important biological characteristic and biological behavior of malignant tumors. Without blocking the cancer cells that are in the process of metastasis, the metastasis of cancer cells cannot be controlled, and it is difficult to obtain the possibility of full cancer treatment. In other words, it is difficult ***to obtain the possibility of cancer treatment for full recovery***.

(4) **According to the cancer cell metastasis pathway, it is to design a new anti-metastasis treatment model to encircle and block**

In summary, cancer treatment includes not only surgical removal of the primary tumor, surgery or radiotherapy or immunochemotherapy for the treatment of metastases for the first two forms, but also the treatment target or target for the third form, that is, to target the cancer cell population on the way of metastasis, to encircle and block the cancer cell population on the way of metastasis, to enhance the host's immune surveillance, and interfere to prevent the metastasis of cancer cells.

According to the metastasis pathway of cancer cells, the metastasis mechanism of multi-step, multi-factor, and multi-link molecular metastasis of cancer cells, new anti-metastatic treatment models are designed, and new treatment methods are designed to intervene and block cancer cells. In other words, it is to design new anti-metastatic treatment models, and new treatment methods to intervene and block cancer cells.

Although there are no clinical manifestations of cancer cells and micrometastasis during metastasis, they do exist.

Only by entering the molecular biology level, gene level, and molecular immune level it can discover and understand these existence, such as the detection of overexpression of various tumor markers, molecular immune gene changes, and micrometastasis, which can now be carried out.

The presence of individual cancer cells (ITC) in the blood and bone marrow can be detected at the molecular level.

New molecular level detection indicators, molecular immune indicators, cytokines, and tumor markers will continue to appear.

It is believed that early diagnosis of precancerous and micro-metastasis will be achieved in the near future.

3. *The process of research and understanding of the third manifestation of cancer in the human body*

(1) Where are the cancer cells during metastasis?

Since it has realized that the key to cancer treatment is anti-metastasis, how to beat against metastasis?

How can it is to understand *the specific process, steps and mechanism about cancer cell metastasis?*

Just like fighting an enemy, how many enemies should be found out?

Where is it?
What's the trend?
How do these cancer cells work or active?
How is its activity pattern?
Where is the weak link of cancer cells in the process of metastasis?
Which link should be cracked down or blocked?

How should the goal of combating cancer metastasis be specific?

(2) **The experimental research to track the fate and law of cancer cells during metastasis**

In order to solve the above-mentioned series of problems, it must conduct basic research on experimental tumors, implement cancer cell transplantation, establish animal models of tumors, and carry out a series of experimental tumor studies:

① Explore the **mechanism and law** of cancer **invasion and metastasis**;

② Discuss **the relationship between tumors and immunity, immune organs**, and **the relationship between immune organs and tumors**:

③ Find the effective measures to regulate and control cancer invasion and metastasis.

The author's laboratory has spent more than 3 years conducting experimental research on animal models of cancer metastasis, as well as experimental *observations to track the fate and laws of cancer cells during metastasis.*

In animal experiments, 10^5 cancer cells were injected intravenously from mice, and no cancer cells were found in the blood after 48 hours.

So who eliminated these injected cancer cells?

The analysis speculates that some cells may not adapt to the environment after being injected into the circulatory system, be damaged by the impact of blood flow, or be obstructed in the microcirculation and be eliminated.

However, most of the cancer cells that enter the blood circulation are mainly eliminated by the mice's own immunity, that is, a large number of immune cells in the mouse blood circulation.

That is, a large number of immune cells in the blood circulation of mice are eliminated by phagocytosis.

Therefore, in anti-metastatic therapy, the treatment of cancer cells and cancer cell populations on the way of metastasis must protect the immunity of the host body, and try to mobilize, restore, and activate the immune function of its immune system.

But It should not or try to avoid hitting, damaging, or reducing the host's immunity and immune system function.

How to protect, mobilize, and activate the host's immune function to deal with cancer cells on the way to metastasis should be an important strategy for anti-metastatic therapy.

(3) *In what form and where the cancer cells on the way of metastasis exist?*

Some new methods have been discovered in animal experiments and some experimental results have been achieved.

However, many experimental results are difficult to pass clinical verification, because clinical verification must be observed for 3-5 years or more to evaluate long-term efficacy.

Often, good results are seen in experimental studies, but it is difficult to observe obvious effects in clinical practice.

Because laboratory research objects are animals and mice, and clinical objects are patients, the experimental results may not always be cited in the clinic.

It must be clinically verified and observed for 3-5 years or even 8-10 years to understand the long-term recurrence and metastasis.

The primary or metastatic lesions of these patients have been treated appropriately or even more satisfactorily.

Why did it happen again in the future or soon, and even spread it widely?

In what form and where do these metastatic and recurring cancer cells exist?

The transfer takes several months or several years. What causes it?

Where are these cancer cells hiding in the human body?

Why is it so stubborn?

As the common people often say: "Cancer is alive and can run", the form of cancer cells in the human body is not only the primary cancer foci and metastases, but there is also a third form, that is, cancer cells and cancer cell populations ***that are on the way to metastasis***.

This third form of expression has not been mentioned in the literature or textbooks so far.

Because people do not know it yet, the special manifestation of cancer cells during metastasis is ignored.

(4) How can cancer cells survive during metastasis?

Although many patients have used a variety of traditional treatment methods, radiotherapy, chemotherapy or comprehensive treatment of primary tumors or metastatic tumors, cancer cells still stubbornly and continuously metastasize.

So where are these cancer cells hiding?

Through research, it is found that the metastasis speed of these cancer cells in the process of metastasis can be fast or slow.

Under certain conditions, sometimes it may be dormant or sleep and stay in the G_0 phase, and sometimes the cancer cells will become active again and enter the cell cycle.

The "condition" mentioned here may be related to the host's immunity, local microenvironment and other factors, or/and it may be related to the cell dynamics of the cancer cells themselves.

These cancer cells in the process of metastasis are the most dangerous "hidden enemy".

Cancer cells with metastatic potential that survive the metastasis process will slowly and gradually form new metastases.

Cancer cells on the way to metastasis survive because they escape the immune surveillance of immune cells in the blood circulation.

If cytotoxic chemotherapy is used to treat metastatic tumors, it may kill too many immune cells, which may further weaken the immune surveillance of immune cells in the patient's blood circulation.

On the contrary, more cancer cells in the process of metastasis escape immune surveillance and form more new metastatic lesions.

4. *Traditional cancer therapy believes that there are two forms*

Traditional cancer therapy believes that there are two manifestations of cancer in the human body:

One is a primary tumor mass,

The other is metastatic nodules or metastases.

The treatment goals or targets of traditional cancer therapy are directed at these two manifestations, namely, primary tumors and metastatic tumors.

Because both primary and metastatic tumors are composed of cancer cells, and the goal of treatment is to kill cancer cells. Traditional therapies mainly rely on surgery, radiotherapy, and chemotherapy to achieve this goal.

The main reasons for the failure of traditional therapies are recurrence and metastasis.

(8) How to do anti-cancer metastasis?

Three steps of anti-cancer metastasis treatment
(Introduction expansion)

1. *It should understand the transfer steps so as to make treatment goals more specific*
2. *Try to defeat ore beat each transfer step one by one*
3. *Three strategies for anti-cancer metastasis treatment("Three Steps")*

1. *It should understand the transfer steps so as to make treatment goals more specific1. Or the transfer steps should be understood to make the treatment goals more specific*

In order to more clearly understand the concept of the extremely complex, dynamic, continuous multi-step, multi-factor biological process of cancer cell metastasis, after the repeated thinking and careful analysis, it is summarized and proposed the "eight steps" of the cancer cell metastasis process.

Based on this "eight steps" theory, it tries to solve the unclear and unspecific concept of understanding the complex biological process of cancer cell metastasis.

In order to carry out scientific design, to intercept or to block and break each transfer step, it is necessary to have a clear and distinct understanding of the concept of each step of the transfer process.

Only when the "target" of each step is clear, it can be maneuverable, and it can study *and explore the prevention and control strategies for each step.*

The previous article has made a detailed elaboration on the three-stage theory of cancer paper cell metastasis.

One of the keys to cancer treatment is how to resist metastasis, and how to scientifically design anti-metastasis is still a bit vague and not specific enough.

People only recognize the seriousness of the harm to patients from transfer, but lack a clear concept and specific effective prevention and control measures. In other words, people only recognize the seriousness of transfer to patients, but lack clear concepts and specific effective *prevention and treatment strategies.*

In order to scientifically design the interception or blocking of each metastasis step, it is designed and formulated about prevention and treatment strategies for each stage based on the eight-step and three-stage theory and the molecular mechanism of cancer cell metastasis, which is called the three-step of anti-cancer metastasis treatment.

2. Try to defeat each transfer step one by one

The basic process of cancer cell metastasis is as the following:

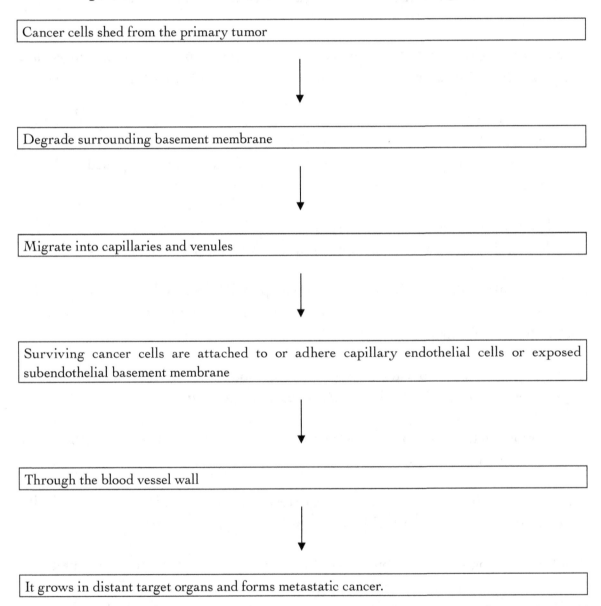

Cancer cells shed from the primary tumor

↓

Degrade surrounding basement membrane

↓

Migrate into capillaries and venules

↓

Surviving cancer cells are attached to or adhere capillary endothelial cells or exposed subendothelial basement membrane

↓

Through the blood vessel wall

↓

It grows in distant target organs and forms metastatic cancer.

This is a ***very complex, dynamic and continuous biological*** process consisting of several relatively independent and interrelated steps.

In each step, a series of molecular biological events will occur between cancer cells and cancer cells, and between cancer cells and host cells, so that the entire metastasis process can be completed and eventually metastatic cancer foci are formed.

In other words, cancer cells must go through each step of the metastasis process to form metastatic cancer foci.

If any step fails, the entire transfer process will stop.

This reminds us that if it tries to break through each step, it will "set the block or stop setting "for the metastatic steps of cancer cells during the metastasis process and implement the strategies and tactics of "encircle, chase, block, and intercept", which may break or block the metastasis pathway and intercept the cancer cells in the metastasis process. In other words, this reminds us that if it tries to break through each step individually, "set cards" for the metastasis steps of cancer cells in the metastasis process, and implement strategies and tactics of "encircle, chase, block, and intercept", it is possible to break or block the way of metastasis so as to intercept cancer cells in the process of metastasis.

__The new concept of cancer treatment and the new model of anti-cancer metastasis treatment are trying to block one or several steps or links of the above-mentioned metastasis process, so as to achieve the purpose of controlling metastasis.__

In order to achieve the above goals, how should it specifically carried out anti-metastasis? What theory will be used? what kind of technology will apply for ? what kind of drug will be used? at which step or stage and link to block cancer cells during metastasis will be?

The following will specifically explain them.

3. *__Three strategies for anti-cancer metastasis treatment ("Three Steps")__*

1). The first step of the anti-cancer is as the following:

1)). Cancer cell metastasis at this stage:

Cancer cells detached from primary cancer

↓

Adhesion to extracellular matrix (ECM)

↓

Degrade ECM and open the way for cancer cells

↓

Cell movement through adhesion and de-adhesion of the degraded matrix

↓

Then reach the outer wall of the blood vessel

↓

Degradation of vascular basement membrane

↓

Do an amoeba-like exercise, first stretch out the pseudofoot

↓

Through the blood vessel wall.

2)). Prevention and control measures:

This stage is the intervention and suppression measures for cancer cells before they break away from the primary tumor and enter the blood vessel.

During this period, the treatment "targets" are mainly anti-adhesion, anti-degradation, anti-movement, and anti-cancer invasion.

3)). *The goal of treatment:*

It prevents cancer cells from entering the blood vessels and achieves the purpose of "beating the enemy outside the country".

2). *The second step of anti-cancer metastasis*

1)). The process of cancer cell metastasis at this stage:

The cancer cell moves through the blood vessel wall into the blood circulation. The detail process is as the following:

Cancer cells are mixed in the blood plasma and various blood cell components, or they are homogeneous adhesion of cancer cells and cancer cells to form a cancer cell population, or heterogeneous adhesions of platelets, white blood cells, etc. to form *tiny tumor thrombi.*

Drifting in the venous system with venous blood flow.

↓

Back to the right heart

↓

Entering the pulmonary artery microcirculation, some cancer cells can park themselves in the pulmonary microcirculation blood vessels (form lung metastases), and some pass through the pulmonary microcirculation.

↓

Enter the pulmonary vein

↓

Back to the left heart

↓

The cancer cells are mixed in the blood flow through the impact force and vortex of the blood flow of the heart valve, and the pump flow enters the aorta and then ejects into the small arteries of various organs.

↓

Enter the microcirculation of various organs and tissues (especially the parenchymal organs, such as liver, kidney, brain and bone cancellous)

↓

Most of the cancer cells in the circulatory journey are damaged by immune cells or by the powerful blood flow impact and shear force, and they die.

A very small number of surviving cancer cells form tiny tumor thrombi, which can adhere to microvascular endothelial cells, degrade the basement membrane, and penetrate outside the blood vessel.

At this stage, cancer cells are floating in the blood circulation, contacting various immune cells, and may be captured and swallowed by various immune cells in the bloodstream, and cannot survive.

A small number of surviving cancer cells escaped immune surveillance in the blood circulation and adhered to vascular endothelial cells.

2)). Prevention countermeasures:

The "target" of anti-metastasis therapy in this phase is to protect and enhance the immune function of various immune cells in the blood circulation, activate immune cytokines and anti-adhesion (homogeneous adhesion between cancer cells and cancer cells, heterogeneous adhesion with platelets, and vascular endothelial Cell adhesion) anti-exercise, anti-platelet aggregation, anti-hypercoagulation, anti-cancer thrombus.

3)). Treatment goals:

It activates immune cells, protects the function of thymus tissue, improves immunity, protects the marrow of blood, and encourages cancer cells floating in the blood circulation to capture, swallow, encircle and block the immune cell population.

The second step is to destroy the main battlefield of cancer cells in the blood circulation drifting movement. It is also the main strategy for intervention and suppression of cancer metastasis.

3). The third step of anti-cancer metastasis

1)). The metastasis of cancer cells at this stage:

Cancer cells evade the surveillance of immune cells in the blood circulation and the killing of immune cells, pass through the blood vessel wall, and anchor to settle in the appropriate organs and tissues in the local microenvironment. The tumors form new microvessels and gradually form metastatic cancer foci.

2)). Prevention and control measures:

To improve *the local microenvironment and tissue immunity*, adjust the local microenvironment, make it unfavorable for the survival and implantation of cancer cells, inhibit angiogenic factors, and inhibit the formation of new blood vessels.

To sum up, the "three steps" of anti-cancer metastasis treatment locates the space for the treatment of cancer metastasis in the blood circulation, and the time is located in three different stages. The emphasis is on improving host immunity.

It can be summarized as the following table and figure below.

Table "Three Steps" of Anti-cancer Metastasis Treatment

Cancer metastasis stage	Transfer through	Prevention countermeasures
The first step of anti-metastasis is in the pre-circulation stage of cancer cell invasion	Separation of cancer cells from primary cancer ↓ Degradation of ECM ↓ Adhesion and de-adhesion ↓ Movement ↓ Before entering the blood vessel	• Anti-adhesion • Anti-degradation • Anti-exercise • Anti-matrix metalloproteinase • Keep cancer cells out of blood vessels
Cancer cells in the blood circulation stage is the anti-metastatic second step	Groups of cancer cells and tiny tumor thrombi float are in the blood circulation, are facing and experiencing the phagocytosis and capture of immune cells and the impact loss of blood flow shear force	• the methods of ani-cancer are to strengthen and activate the various immune cells and factors in the circulation, to enhance the immune function, and the circulation system is the main battlefield for annihilating cancer cells on the way to metastasis. • Anti-adhesion • Anti-platelet aggregation • Anticancer thrombus

That cancer cells escape the bleeding cycle and anchor the "target" organ tissue stage is the third step of anti-metastasis	After the cancer cells escape from the blood vessels, they anchor the "target" organs and tissues, and new blood vessels form and metastases are formed.	• TC • Inhibit angiogenesis factor • Inhibit blood vessel formation • Increase immune regulation • Improve local microenvironmental tissue immunity

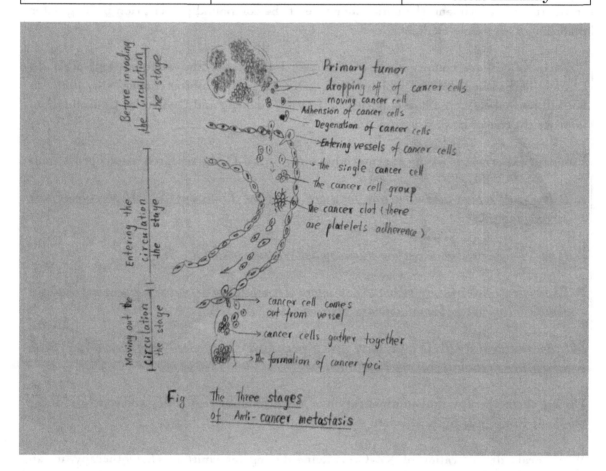

Pre-invasion cycle/Primary tumor/Shed cancer cells/Stick(adherence)/ Degradation of ECM/ Sports(movement)/Cancer cells penetrate blood vessels/ Post-invasion stage/Single cancer cell/Cancer cell population/Cancer thrombus (with platelet adhesion)/Cancer cells pass through blood vessels

Post-vascularization/Cancer cell aggregation/Metastasis formation

Figure three stages of anti-cancer metastasis

(9)   The methods and drugs of Cancer Treatment

(Introduction Expansion)

Overview

XZ-C immune regulatory and control anti-cancer Chinese medicine is 48 kinds of Chinese herbal medicines with good tumor inhibition rates which have been screened through tumor suppression experiments in cancer-bearing mice.

In the tumor experiment, the anti-tumor rate of the compound prescription is far greater than that of the single-medicine.

XZ-C1, XZ-C4 are compromised of Shencao, Longyacao, Shuyangquan and other 28 Chinese herbal medicines, of which XZ-C$_{1-A}$, XZ-C$_{1-B}$ 100% inhibit cancer cells, 100% do not kill normal cells, and have a positive effect for Fuzheng and Guoben or Consolidation, improve the role of human immune function.

From our experiments on the pharmacodynamics of XZ-C, the research results prove that:

1. *It has good tumor inhibition rate for Ehrlich ascites carcinoma, S_{180}, H_{22} hepatocellular carcinoma;*

2. *It has obvious effect of increasing efficiency and reducing toxicity;*

3. *Experiments have also proved that XZ-C immune regulation and control Chinese medicine can significantly improve human immune function.*

After the acute toxicity test in mice, there is no obvious toxic side effects, and no obvious side effects have been seen in clinical oral administration for several years (2-6 years).

During chemotherapy, oral administration of XZ-C immune regulatory and control chinese medicine can significantly alleviate side effects.

While oral administration of XZ-C medicine during intermittent chemotherapy, it can increase white blood cells and increase hemoglobin.

Most advanced cancer patients have weakness, fatigue, and loss of appetite. After 4-8-12 weeks of taking XZ-C immunomodulatory anti-cancer medicine, they can significantly improve appetite, sleep, relieve pain, and gradually restore physical strength.

The experimental research and clinical verification work has been carried out.

A.   <u>The experimental research work</u>

Our laboratory has carried out the following experimental studies to screen the new anti-cancer and anti-metastatic drugs from Chinese medication:

1. In vitro screening test:

Use cancer cell culture in vitro to observe the direct damage of cancer cell drugs to cancer cells.

Put crude drug powder products (500ug/ml) into the test tubes for culturing cancer cells to observe whether they have an inhibitory effect on cancer paper cells and their tumor inhibition rate.

2. In vivo tumor suppression screening test:

To create a cancer-bearing animal model and conduct an experimental screening study on the anti-cancer rate of Chinese herbal medicines in cancer-bearing animals.

Each batch of experiments uses 240 mice, divided into 8 experimental groups, each with 30 rats, the seventh group is the blank control group, 8 groups used 5-Fu or CTX as the control group.

All mice were inoculated with EAC or S_{180} or H_{22} cancer cells,

After 24 hours of inoculation, each mouse was orally fed with crude and raw drug powder, and the selected traditional Chinese medicine was fed for a long time. The survival period was observed and the tumor inhibition rate was calculated.

In this way, we have conducted experimental research for 4 consecutive years, using more than 1,000 tumor-bearing animal models each year, and a total of nearly 6,000 tumor-bearing animal models have been made in 4 years.

After the death of each experimental mouse, pathological anatomy of ***liver, spleen, lung, thymus, and kidney*** was performed, and more than 20,000 tissue slide or resections were performed.

3. The experimental results:

Among the 200 Chinese herbal medicines screened by animal experiments in our laboratory, 48 kinds of Chinese herbal medicines were screened to have certain or even excellent inhibitory effects on cancer cells, with a tumor inhibition rate of over 75-90%.

This group has been screened by animal experiments and eliminated 152 species without obvious anticancer effects.

B. Clinical validation

It is to perform clinical verification on the basis of successful animal experiments.

1. Method:

a. It was to establish an oncology specialist outpatient clinic and the scientific research team with an integrated Chinese and Western medicine anti-cancer, anti-metastasis, and anti-recurrence.

b. It was to keep outpatient medical records.

c. It was to establish a complete follow-up observation system.

d. It was to observe the long-term effect.

e. It was from experimental research to clinical verification, when new problems are discovered in the clinical verification process, they return to the laboratory for basic research, and then apply the new experimental results to the clinic.

So, it is to form the model:

It is from the experiment to the clinical to re-experiment to re-clinical.

In brief, the experimental research must pass clinical verification.

A large number of patients have been observed for 3-5 years or even 8-10 years.

According to evidence-based medicine, there are long-term follow-up and evaluable data.

The efficacy criteria are:
The quality of life is good and the life span is long.

The result is:

XZ-C immunomodulatory anti-cancer Chinese medicine preparations have been applied and observed by a large number of patients with advanced cancer, and have achieved remarkable effects.

2. <u>Clinical data:</u>

The anticancer Research Cooperation Group with combination of Chinese and Western Medicine and Shuguang Oncology Specialty Outpatient Department used XZ-C immunomodulatory anticancer Chinese medicine to treat 4698 cases of stage III, IV or metastatic or recurrent cancer, including 3051 males and 1647 females, the youngest 11 years old, up to 86 years old, all patients in the group were diagnosed with pathological slices or CT, MRI, and B-ultrasound imaging.

According to the International Anti-Cancer Alliance's staging standards, all cases were stage III or higher, including:

1021 cases of liver cancer,

752 cases of lung cancer,

694 cases of gastric cancer,

624 cases of esophageal and cardia cancer,

326 cases of rectal cancer,

442 cases of colon cancer, and 368 cases of breast cancer,

74 cases of pancreatic cancer,

30 cases of bile duct cancer,

43 cases of retroperitoneal tumors,

38 cases of ovarian cancer,

9 cases of cervical cancer,

11 cases of brain tumors,

34 cases of thyroid cancer,

38 cases of nasopharyngeal carcinoma, and 9 cases of melanoma,

27 cases of kidney cancer,

48 cases of bladder cancer,

13 cases of leukemia,

47 cases of supraclavicular metastasis,

35 cases of various sarcomas,

39 cases of other malignant tumors.

3. <u>Drugs and methods of administration:</u>

<u>*The treatment principle is to protect the thymus and increase immune function, and protect bone marrow and promote blood production, thereby enhancing the host's immune surveillance and controlling the immune escape of cancer cells.*</u>

<u>*From the perspective of traditional Chinese medication, the treatment is to strengthen the body and eliminate the evil, or to support the rightness and remove the damage; soften the firmness and dispel or dissolve lumps, and to supplement tonic the qi and blood.*</u>

The drugs are $XZ-C_1$, $XZ-C_2$, $XZ-C_3$, $XZ-C_4$, $XZ-C_5$, $XZ-C_6$, $XZ-C_7$, $XZ-C_8$, ------$XZ-C_{10}$.

Depending on different cancers and disease conditions, metastasis situation; according to the dialectical condition, it is to choose the above drugs.

For solid tumors or metastatic masses, all of them are to take anti-cancer medication internally or anticancer powder orally and anticancer antitumor ointment for external use.

Anticancer analgesic ointment should be used for painful patients.

Tuihuangtang or Xiaoshuitang should be used for jaundice and ascites.

4. **The treatment results:**

The symptoms are improved, the quality of life is improved, and the survival period is prolonged.

(1) Among 4277 patients with advanced cancer who took XZ-C$_{1-10}$ immunomodulatory Chinese medicine for more than 3 months, the medical records have detailed curative effect observation records, see the table below.

Table. Observation of 4277 Cases of Curative Effect on comprehensively Improvement of the Quality of Life of Patients with Advanced Cancer

Improvement	spirit	appetite	Strengthen	General conditions improve	Weight gain	Sleep better	Improvement activities Ability activity Limited relief	Self-care Walking activity usual	Return to work Doing light work Number of cases
Case	4071	3986	2450	479	2938	1005	1038	3220	479
(%)	95.2	93.2	57.3	11.2	68.7	23.5	24. 3	75.3	11. 2

All patients in this group are in the middle and late stages, and all have different degrees of symptom improvement after taking the medicine, with an effective rate of 93.2%.

In terms of improving the quality of life (according to the Karnofsky scoring standard), the average score is 50 before the medication, and the average is increased to 80 after the medication. The patients in this group have metastasis and dysfunction of different tissues and organs above stage III.

Past statistics of such patients is reported that the median survival time is about 6 months. The longest cases in this group have reached 18 years, and the average survival time of the She cases is more than 1 year.

a. One case of primary liver cancer in the left lobe of the liver, recurred in the right liver after resection, and had been treated with XZ-C medicine for 18 years;

b. Another case of liver cancer has been taking XZ-C for 10 and a half years;

c. In 2 cases of liver cancer, there were multiple tumors in the liver. After taking XZ-C for half a year, the tumors completely disappeared after 2 CT re-examinations, and they have been stable for half a year;

d. 1 case of double kidney cancer, extensive metastasis to the abdominal cavity after one side resection, after taking XZ-C medicine, has completely returned to work;

e. 3 cases of lung cancer could not be cut through open chest examination. Long-term use of XZ-C drug has been 3 and a half years;

f. 2 cases of remnant gastric cancer took XZ-C medicine for 8 years;

g. 3 cases of rectal cancer recurrence have been taking XZ-C medicine for 3 years;

h. 1 case of breast cancer metastasis to liver and ribs has been taking medicine for 8 years;

i. 1 female patient with a walnut-sized lymph node mass in both groin and neck was diagnosed as non-Hodgkin's lymphoma by pathology. She could not undergo chemotherapy due to financial difficulties. She took $XZ\text{-}C_1 + XZ\text{-}C_4 + XZ\text{-}C_2$ in 2015, I came to the outpatient clinic for follow-up visits every month, and the condition was generally good.

j. 1 case of recurrence of bladder cancer after renal cancer surgery, taking XZ-C drug for 9 and a half years;

The above cases are all patients in the middle and advanced stages who cannot undergo surgery, radiotherapy, or chemotherapy. ***They are treated with ZX-C drugs only and no other drugs are used.***

So far, I still come to the clinic every month for review and medicine. After taking the medicine for a long time, the condition is controlled in a stable state, so that the body and the tumor are in a balanced state for a long time, and a better survival with the tumor is obtained. The patient's condition is improved, the quality of life is improved, and the survival period is prolonged.

(2) For 84 cases of solid tumors and 56 cases of patients with metastatic supraclavicular lymphadenopathy, it was to achieve better results with the internal application of XZ-C series and external ointment application of XZ-C anti-cancer lighting harden knot, see the table below:

Table. Changes of 84 cases of solid tumors and 56 cases of metastatic nodules after external application of XZ-C ointment

	Solid tumor mass				Swollen supraclavicular lymph nodes in the neck			
	Disappear	Reduce ½	Turn soft	No change	Disappear	Reduce ½	Turn soft	No change
Case	12	28	32	12	12	22	14	8
(%)	14.2	33.3	38.0	14.2	21.4	39.2	25.0	14.2
Total effective rate (%)	85.7				85.7			

298 patients with cancer pain achieved significant pain relief after oral administration of XZ-C medicine and external application of XZ-C anticancer pain relief ointment. See the table below.

Table of pain relief after oral administration of XZ-C drug and external application of XZ-C anticancer pain relief ointment in 298 patients

Clinical manifestations	Pain			
	Mild relief	Significantly reduced	Disappear	Invalid
Number of cases (%)	52	139	93	14
	17.3	46.8	31.2	4.7
Total effective rate (%)	95.3%			

5. Exclusive scientific research products:

The series products of XZ-C immune regulation and control of anti-cancer Chinese medicine

(introduction)

The series of traditional Chinese medicine preparations of the self-developed XZ-C (XU ZE China) immune-regulated and controlled anti-cancer, from experimental research to clinical verification, have been applied to clinical practice on the basis of successful animal experiments. After many years of clinical cases Clinically verified, the effect is remarkable. It is the result of independent invention, independent innovation and independent intellectual property rights.

Research on finding and screening new anti-cancer and anti-metastasis drugs from traditional Chinese medicine:

The purpose is to screen out anti-cancer, anti-metastasis, and anti-relapse intelligent anti-cancer drugs that have no drug resistance, no toxic side effects, high selectivity, and long-term oral administration.

It is well known that the anticancer agents currently used in the world can indeed inhibit the proliferation of cancer paper cells, but they kill both cancer cells and normal cells, especially bone marrow immune cells, and severely damage the host, because cytotoxic drugs of the chemotherapy line are not selective.

Moreover, traditional chemotherapy suppresses immune function and suppresses bone marrow hematopoietic function. Traditional intravenous chemotherapy is an intermittent treatment, the interstitial phase cannot be treated, and the interstitial phase cancer cells continue to proliferate and divide. Although chemotherapeutics can inhibit the proliferation of cancer cells, when the cancer has not been eliminated, the drug has to be stopped due to its side effects. After stopping the drug, the cancer cells proliferated again and began to have drug resistance. When resistance develops, this dose will not work, so increase the dose. However, if the dose is increased, it may endanger the patient's life. If the given chemotherapeutic drug has drug resistance, it will not only have no effect on cancer cells, but will only kill the patient's normal cells.

Therefore, cancer cells are resistant to anticancer drugs and the toxic side effects of anticancer drugs on the host It is a long-term troublesome problem. **The purpose of the new drugs we are looking for is to avoid these shortcomings.**

According to the theory of cell proliferation cycle, the anticancer agent must be able to be applied continuously for a long time, so that the cancer focus can be continuously immersed in the anticancer agent for a long time, so as to prevent its cell division and prevent recurrence and metastasis.

It must be carried out over a long period of time, and it is best to take medicine for a long time to control the existing cancer foci and prevent the formation of new cancer cells. However, the currently used anticancer drugs cannot be used continuously for a long period of time due to the large side effects. Existing anticancer drugs all have the side effects of suppressing immune function, suppressing hematopoietic function of bone marrow, suppressing thymus, and suppressing bone marrow.

The formation and development of cancer is because the patient's immunity is reduced and the immune monitoring is lost. Therefore, all anti-cancer drugs should increase immunity and protect immune organs, and should not use drugs that suppress immunity.

To this end, our laboratory has carried out the following experimental studies to screen the new anti-cancer and anti-metastatic drugs from Chinese medicine:

(A) *Using the method of in vitro culturing of cancer cells, the screening experiment study of Chinese herbal medicine anti-tumor rate:*

In vitro screening test:

The cancer cells are cultured in vitro to observe the direct damage of the drugs to the cancer cells.

In the test tube screening test, put crude drugs (500ug/ml) into the test tubes for culturing cancer cells to observe whether they have inhibitory effects on cancer cells. We take 200 kinds of Chinese herbal medicines that traditional Chinese medicine thinks have anti-cancer effects to perform one by one in vitro screening test. They were cultured with normal fibroblasts under the same conditions to test the toxicity of the drug to such cells and then compare them.

(B) *Manufacture of cancer-bearing animal models, and conduct experimental screening research on the anti-cancer rate of Chinese herbal medicine in cancer-bearing animals*

In vivo cancer suppression screening test

Each batch of experiment uses 240 mice, divided into 8 groups, each group has 30 mice, the 7th group is the blank control group, the 8th group uses 5-Fu or CTX as the control group, the whole group of mice is inoculated with EAC or S_{180} or H_{22} cancer cell.

After 24 hours of inoculation, each mouse was orally fed with crude crude drug powder, and fed with the selected traditional Chinese medicine for a long time to observe the survival period, toxicity and side effects, calculate the prolonged survival rate, and calculate the tumor suppression rate.

In this way, we conducted 4 consecutive years of experimental research, and also conducted 3 years of experimental research on the pathogenesis, metastasis and recurrence mechanisms of tumor-bearing mice, as well as experimental research to **explore why tumors cause the death of the host.** More than 1,000 tumor-bearing animal models are used every year, and nearly 6,000 tumor-bearing animal models have been made in 4 years.

After the death of each experimental mouse, pathological anatomy of the liver, spleen, lung, thymus, and kidney was performed, and more than 20,000 sections or slides were performed to explore whether there may be micro-pathogens that may cause cancer.

Microcirculation microscope was used to observe tumor microvascular establishment and microcirculation in 100 tumor-bearing mice.

Through experimental research, we discovered for the first time in China that the traditional Chinese medicine TG has a significant effect on inhibiting tumor microvessel formation. It has been used in clinical anti-metastasis treatment for more than 80 patients, and the effect is being observed.

The Experimental results:

Among the 200 Chinese herbal medicines screened in our laboratory through animal experiments, 48 kinds of Chinese herbal medicines were screened to have certain or even excellent inhibitory effects on the proliferation of cancer cells, and the tumor inhibition rate was above 75-90%.

However, there are also some commonly used Chinese medicines that are generally considered to have anti-cancer effects. They have no anti-cancer effects after screening in vitro and in vivo tumor inhibition rates, or have little effect. This group has been screened and eliminated by animal experiments to eliminate 152 types without obvious anti-cancer effects.

The 48 traditional Chinese medicines with good tumor suppression rate selected from this experiment were optimized and combined to repeat the tumor suppression rate test in the cancer-bearing body.

__Finally, the XU ZE China1-10 preparation (XZ-C1-10), an immune-regulating anti-cancer traditional Chinese medicine with Chinese characteristics was developed.__

XZ-C1 can obviously inhibit cancer cells, but does not affect normal cells;

XZ-C4 can promote thymus hyperplasia and increase immunity;

XZ-C8 can protect the blood of the marrow and protect the hematopoietic function of bone marrow.

The clinical verification is carried out on the basis of successful animal experiments. That is,

1). to establish an oncology specialist outpatient clinic and a combined anti-cancer, anti-metastasis, and recurrence scientific research team;

2). keep outpatient medical records;

3). establish a regular follow-up observation system;

4). and observe long-term treatment effects.

5). From the experimental research to the clinical verification, the new problems were discovered in the clinical verification process, and then returned to the laboratory for basic research, and then applied the new experimental results to clinical verification.

In this way, the experiment ------the clinical ------the re-experiment ------the re-clinical, all experimental research must pass clinical verification, observe on a large number of patients for 3-5 years, even clinical observation for 8-10 years, according to evidence-based medicine, there are long-term follow-up and evaluable data which to make sure that it clearly and indeed has a good long-term curative effect.

The standard of curative effect is:

The quality of life is good and the life span is long.

XZ-C immunomodulatory anti-cancer Chinese medicine preparations have been validated by a large number of patients with advanced cancer and have achieved remarkable results.

XZ-C immune regulation and control Chinese medication can improve the quality of life of patients with advanced cancer, enhance immunity, increase the body's anti-cancer ability, increase appetite, and significantly prolong survival.

The introduction is as follows:

(1) *The Study on the mechanism of XZ-C immune regulation and control anti-cancer Chinese medication*

With the continuous deepening of research on traditional Chinese medicine, many traditional Chinese medicines are known to have regulatory effects on the production and biological activities of cytokines and other immune molecules.

At this time, it is of great significance to elucidate the immunological mechanism of XZ-C immune regulation and anti-cancer Chinese medicine *at the molecular level.*

1). XZ-C anti-cancer Chinese medicine can protect immune organs and increase the *weight of thymus and spleen*.

2) XZ-C anti-cancer Chinese medicine has obvious promoting effect on *bone marrow cell proliferation and hematopoietic* function.

3). XZ-C anti-cancer traditional Chinese medicine can enhance the *immune function of T cells*, and has a significant proliferation effect on T cells.

4). XZ-C anti-cancer traditional Chinese medicine can significantly enhance the production of human IL-2.

5). XZ-C anti-cancer Chinese medicine can activate and enhance the activity of NK cells. NK cells have a broad-spectrum anti-tumor effect and can kill xenogeneic tumor cells.

6). XZ-C anti-cancer Chinese medicine can enhance the activity of LAK cells.

LAK cells can kill solid elbow tumor cells that are sensitive and insensitive to NK cells, and have a broad-spectrum anti-tumor effect.

7). XZ-C anti-cancer Chinese medicine can induce and promote the induction of interferon(IFN).

IFN has broad-spectrum anti-tumor and immunomodulatory effects.

IFN can inhibit tumor cell proliferation.

IFN can activate NK cells and CTL to kill tumor cells..

8). XZ-C anti-cancer Chinese medicine can promote and enhance colony stimulating factors (CSF).

CSF not only participates in the proliferation and differentiation of hematopoietic cells, but also plays an important role in the host's anti-tumor immunity.

9). XZ-C anti-cancer Chinese medicine has the effect of promoting tumor necrosis factor (TNF).

TNF is a type of cytokine that can directly cause tumor cell death, and its main biological function is to kill or inhibit tumor cells.

(1) *Biological response modifier (BRM) and BRM-like Chinese medicine and tumor treatment*

1)). *Biological response modifiers (BRM) have opened up a new field of tumor biotherapy. At present, BRM, as the fourth program of tumor treatment, has received extensive attention from the medical community.*

In 1982, Oldharn founded the biological response modifier (BRM) or BRM theory. On this basis, the family proposed the fourth modality of cancer treatment (four modality of cancer treatment)-biological treatment in 1984.

According to the BRM theory, under normal circumstances, the tumor and the body's defense are in a dynamic balance.

The occurrence, invasion and metastasis of tumors are completely caused by the imbalance of this dynamic balance.

If the disordered state is artificially adjusted to a normal level, the growth of the tumor can be controlled and the tumor can be regressed.

Specifically, BRM includes the following anti-tumor mechanisms:

① *Promote the enhancement of the effect of the host defense mechanism, or reduce the immunosuppression of the tumor-bearing soil, so as to achieve the ability of immune response to cancer.*

② *Inject natural or genetically recombined biologically active substances to enhance the host's defense mechanism.*

③ *Modify tumor cells to induce strong host response.*

④ *Promote the differentiation and maturation of tumor cells and make them normalized.*

⑤ *Reduce the side effects of cancer chemotherapy and radiotherapy, and enhance the tolerance of the host.*

2)). *The BRM-like effect and curative effect of XZ-C immune regulation and anticancer Chinese medications*

XZ-C immunomodulatory anti-cancer traditional Chinese medicine has undergone 4 years of cancer-bearing animal experimental research and 10 years of clinical verification to show that it has a BRM-like effect and curative effect. It is a drug with BRM-like effect that has been screened and unearthed from Chinese medicine resources.

XZ-C Immune Control Anti-cancer Chinese Medicine was selected by Professor Xu Ze's laboratory from 200 Chinese herbal medicines.

Firstly, the cancer cells were cultured in vitro, and 200 Chinese herbal medicines were screened one by one in vitro, and the experimental study on the direct damage of each drug to the cancer cells in the culture tube was observed.

And it took the chemotherapy drug CTX and test tube cultured normal cells as the control group to compare the tumor inhibition rate.

As a result, a batch of drugs that have a certain inhibitory rate on cancer cell proliferation were selected.

Then further create tumor-bearing animal models, carry out experimental research on the in vivo tumor inhibition rate screening of tumor-bearing animal models on 200 kinds of Chinese herbal medicines, and carry out scientific, objective and rigorous experimental screening, analysis, and evaluation.

The experimental results showed as the followings:

The experiment proved that only 48 kinds of Chinese herbal medicines have good tumor inhibition rate, and the other 152 common Chinese herbal medicines have been screened by the tumor inhibition rate in this group of tumor-bearing experiments, which proves that there is no anti-cancer effect or the tumor inhibition rate is very low.

The XZ-C immunomodulatory anti-cancer metastasis Chinese medicine screened out through the above experiment does have a good tumor inhibition rate.

It can improve immunity, increase thymus weight, protect thymic tissue function, improve cellular immunity, promote bone marrow cell proliferation, and protect bone marrow blood function, increase the number of red blood cells and white blood cells, enhance T cell function, activate immune cytokines, and improve the immune surveillance effect in the bloodstream.

The main pharmacological effect of XZ-C immune regulation and anti-cancer Chinese medicine is anti-cancer promotion, and its anti-cancer mechanism is:

① **Activate the body's immune cell system, promote the enhancement of the effect of the host's defense mechanism, and achieve the ability of immune response to cancer.**

② **Activate the immune cytokine system of the body's anti-cancer mechanism, enhance the host's defense mechanism and improve the immune surveillance of immune cells in the body's blood circulation system.**

③ **Protect Thymus and promote immunity, increase immunity, protect the marrow to produce blood, protect the bone marrow hematopoietic function, stimulate the bone marrow hematopoietic function, promote the recovery of bone marrow suppression, and increase white blood cells and red blood cells.**

④ **Reducing the side effects of radiotherapy and chemotherapy and enhancing the tolerance of the host.**

⑤ It can increase the weight of the thymus, so that the thymus does not shrink progressively, because the thymus gland progressively shrinks when the cancer progresses.

As mentioned above, the mechanism of action of XZ-C immunoregulatory anti-cancer Chinese medicine is basically similar to that of BRM, and the same therapeutic effect of BRM can be obtained in clinical use.

Therefore, XZ-C immunomodulatory anti-cancer Chinese medicine has BRM-like effects and curative effects. It combines current advanced molecular oncology theories with ancient Chinese herbal medicine resources at the molecular level of Chinese and Western medicine, and use BRM theory as a bridge to connect with advanced international modern molecular oncology theories and practices.

(1) XZ-C1 "Smart Anti-Cancer"

A. *The main ingredients:*

The eight taste anticancer medications

B *The anticancer Pharmacology*

1. Clearing heat and detoxification, invigorating blood circulation and removing blood stasis, strengthening the body, removing evil without hurting the body, strongly inhibits cancer cells, inhibits cancer cell metastasis, and does not inhibit normal cells.

2. In vivo anti-cancer test in mice, it has inhibitory activity on mouse Ehrlich ascites cancer cells, and there is a significant difference between the administration group and the control group.

3. It can prolong the survival time of mice bearing cancer and increase the survival rate of mice by 26.92%.

4. The main drugs XZ-C1-A and XZ-C1-B in the prescription have stable and significant anti-cancer effects, inhibiting cancer cells by 100%, the mitotic phase of cancer cells in the administration group is reduced, and degeneration and necrosis are serious.

It has no effect on epithelial cells or fiber cells.

The water extract of XZ-C1-D in the prescription has inhibitory activity on human cervical cancer cells, and the inhibition rate of mouse sarcoma S180 is as high as 98.9%. The other flavors in the prescription also have strong anticancer effects.

5. The anti-tumor effect of XZ-C1 Chinese medicine on H22 mice bearing liver cancer:

The tumor inhibition rate of XZ-C1 was 40% in the second week, 45% in the 4th week, and 58% in the 6th week.

In the control group, the tumor inhibition rate was 45% in the second week after CTX medication.

The tumor inhibition rate was 45% in the 4th week and 49% in the 6th week.

6. The effect of XZ-C1 Chinese medicine on the survival period of H22-bearing mice:

The life extension rate of the XZ-C1 group was 85%, and the life extension rate of the CTX control group (the chemotherapy drug cyclophosphamide) was 9.8%,

The thymus in the XZ-C1 treatment group did not shrink, while the thymus in the control group shrank significantly.

C. *The clinical application*

1. The indications:

Esophageal cancer, stomach cancer, colorectal cancer, lung cancer, breast cancer, liver cancer, bile duct cancer, pancreatic cancer, thyroid cancer, nasopharyngeal cancer, brain tumor, kidney cancer, bladder cancer, ovarian cancer, cervical cancer, various sarcomas and Various metastatic and recurrent cancers.

2. The usage:

XZ-C1 feels effective after taking 1-3 months continuously,

It can be taken for a long time, one dose every other day after three years, and two doses a week after five years to keep the immune function and cytokines at a certain level for a long time.

D. *The toxicity test*

XZ-Cl can be taken for a long time. Acute toxicity experiments show that mice were gavaged at 104 times the adult dose (10g/Kg body weight). It is to observe at 24, 48, 72, and 96 hours respectively, none of the 30 purebred mice death.

LD50 is difficult to make, and it is a fairly safe prescription.

It has been used in this cancer specialist clinic for many years. Some patients in the clinic have been taking it for 3-5 years for a long time, and it can also be taken for 8-10 years to maintain the body's immunity and prevent recurrence and metastasis. This prescription can be taken for a long time and is quite a safe oral anticancer drug.

(2)   XZ-C2

A. *The main ingredients*

Nine-flavored anti-cancer medicine

A. *The anticancer Pharmacology*

1. Animal experiments can prolong the survival period of L7212 mice (leukemia mice), which is statistically significant compared with the control group.

2. It can increase the inhibition rate of L7212 mice

3. XZ-C2-A and XZ-C2-B have a strong inhibitory effect on mouse sarcoma (S 180).

C. *The clinical application*

The indications:

1. Leukemia, upper gastrointestinal cancer, tongue cancer, laryngeal cancer, nasopharyngeal cancer, esophageal cancer, cervical cancer, bone metastasis.

2. Recurrence of anastomotic stenosis after esophageal cancer or gastric cancer (for those who cannot be operated on).

3. The effect on acute lymphocytic leukemia is general, and it has obvious effect on other types of leukemia.

4. It has a significant effect on the control of bone metastasis.

How to use this medication? Or The usage:

Generally it can be used as 1 capsule Qid or 2 capsules tid;

For Leukemia, it can be used as 3 capsules tid after meal, 7 days as a course of treatment.

(3) XZ-C3 Aitong Powder for external application of acupoints

A. *The main ingredients*

Fifteen tastes or items Anticancer Drugs

B. *The anticancer Pharmacology*

1. To clear away heat and detoxify, relieve inflammation and relieve pain, regulate qi and relieve pain;

2. Promoting blood circulation and removing addiction, reducing swelling and pain, altogether has the effects of clearing away heat and toxins, reducing swelling and pain, and the above-mentioned **analgesic effects are the most prominent.**

3. It is suitable for acupoint application, which can exert the medicine effect better than simply applying the painful area and achieve the purpose of rapid pain relief.

C. *The prescription contents*

The basic recipe: 14 flavors such as sana and turmeric

D. *The clinical application*

Indications:

Liver cancer, lung cancer pain, pancreatic cancer back pain, bone cancer pain points, neck and supraclavicular metastatic lymph node masses.

The usage:

Take an appropriate amount of honey to mix with the powder medications, and stir evenly into a paste for later use.

Apply it to the Rugen acupoint (the 5th and 6th intercostal spaces under the nipple straight down) for lung cancer, and apply to Qimen acupoint for liver cancer (6-7 intercostal spaces in the midline of the breast).

After the medicine, cover with gauze and fix with tape.

For severe pain, change it once in 6 hours, and change it once in 12 hours for mild pain.

Use it continuously until the pain is relieved or disappeared.

The Experience:

Treatment of 84 patients with liver cancer and lung cancer pain has an analgesic effect.

Generally, with 3 times of medication, the pain can be relieved to varying degrees.

After 3-7 days, there is obvious analgesic effect, and some are basically analgesic.

(4) XZ-C4 Thymus Protector and Increasing Immune function (AiKangsan) (5g/bag)

A. The main ingredients

Twelve flavours precious Chinese herbal medicine

B. The anticancer Pharmacology

1. Promote the transformation of lymphocytes, enhance cellular immune function, increase white blood cells, inhibit cancer cells, and warm blood and support gas.

2. Ehrlich ascites cancer cells were transplanted into the abdominal cavity of mice. Chemotherapy drugs were given to mice twice on the first and seventh days after transplantation. At the same time, taking XZ-C4 (2g/kg) daily can significantly enhance the efficacy of chemotherapy drugs.

3. When MMC is used as a chemotherapy drug, it can inhibit the white blood cell decline and weight loss caused by MMC.

4. Anti-cancer chemical drugs were injected into the vein of cancer-bearing mice while taking XZ-C4. It was found that the effect of inhibiting cancer cells was more than three times higher than that of chemotherapy alone.

5. Chemotherapeutics damage the immune organs such as the thymus and spleen of cancer-bearing mice, but after the addition of XZ-C4, the thymus, spleen and other organs do not shrink at all, indicating that XZ-C4 has a protective effect on immune organs.

6. After the XZ-C4 extract of Ehrlich ascites cancer mice was given, the life extension rate of mice was as high as 167.1%, and the average survival time of mice in the control group was 15.2 days, while the XZ-C4 administration group was 25.4 days, it also showed that the function of the mouse reticuloendothelial system was significantly improved.

7. XZ-C4 can quickly reduce the side effects of the chemotherapy drug cisplatin and improve the efficacy of cisplatin.

XZ-C4 can 100% inhibit the toxic and side effects of cisplatin, and the dosage is the normal daily amount of humans.

XZ-C4 does not resist the cancer resistance of cisplatin.

XZ-C4 can protect the kidneys, so that the renal damage of cisplatin hardly occurs.

XZ-C4 is a promising anti-cancer powder clinically.

8. XZ-C4 has a significant effect on patients after cancer surgery. After radical resection of gastrointestinal, hepatopancreatic and other cancers, they all manifested as decreased physical strength, decreased immunity, fatigue, loss of appetite and anemia, etc.

Within 1-2 weeks after surgery, starting from being able to take oral or gastric tube feeding, oral XZ-C4 granules, 7.5 grams per day, 3 times before meals, treatment for 12 weeks, during which chemotherapy or immunotherapy can be performed.

9. XZ-C4 Traditional Chinese Medicine's anti-tumor effect on H22 mice bearing liver cancer:

The tumor inhibition rate of XZ-C4 was 55% in the second week, 68% in the fourth week, and 70% in the sixth week;

In the control group, the tumor inhibition rate of CTX (cyclophosphamide) was 45% in the second week and 49% in the fourth week.

10. The effect of XZ-C4 Chinese medicine on the survival time of H22 mice bearing liver cancer. The survival rate of XZ-C4 group was 200%, and that of CTX group was 9.8%.

11. XZ-C4 can significantly improve immune function, increase white blood cells and red blood cells, have no effect on liver and kidney functions, and have no damage to liver and kidney slices.

CTX reduces white blood cells and reduces immune function. Kidney slices have kidney damage.

12. The thymus in the XZ-C treatment group did not shrink and was slightly enlarged, while the thymus in the CTX control group was significantly atrophied. XZ-C4 has a strong inhibitory effect on mouse sarcoma (S180).

C. The clinical application

1. The indications are the followings:

Various cancers, sarcomas, various advanced cancers, metastatic and recurrent cancers, adjuvant radiotherapy, chemotherapy, and post-surgery patients. It can be used for all kinds of cancer, especially for dizziness, fatigue, fatigue, lazy speech, lack of qi, spontaneous sweating, palpitations, insomnia, and deficiency of both qi and blood.

XZ-C4 immunomodulation Chinese medicine, start to take the medicine before surgery and do clinical and laboratory examination every 4 weeks after taking the medicine, lasting 20 weeks.

The Checking items are the following:

Conscious and objective symptoms, body weight, total protein and albumin, total cholesterol, dielectric, ALL, AST blood routine and the number of platelets, lymphocytes, T cells and B cells, r globulin, urine protein.

The treatment results are the followings:

1. The number of lymphocytes has increased, which can inhibit leukopenia;

2. No effect on liver function;

3. It protects the kidneys and does not damage the kidneys

4. It can significantly reduce skin rashes and stomatitis caused by chemotherapy and radiotherapy;

5. Effective for recovery of physical strength after surgery, chemotherapy and radiotherapy, it can increase appetite, improve body fatigue and gain weight.

XZ-C4 reduces the side effects of radiotherapy and chemotherapy and improves the overall condition of patients after surgery. It is a rare healing medicine.

The Experiences:

Modern medicine has proposed a variety of treatment methods for advanced cancer, but there are still some problems. It is not yet certain whether the combined use of chemotherapy drugs for advanced cancer will be effective.

Even if it is effective, it also brings serious toxic and side effects. It can be considered that the treatment of cancer in modern medicine is to kill cancer cells and is aggressive, while Chinese medicine strengthens the body's own regulatory function to control and even eliminate cancer.

For this reason, it is necessary to find a treatment method that reduces or eliminates symptoms, makes the disease better or treats, has fewer side effects, and can prolong life. XZ-C4 has such characteristics and advantages.

Through experiments XZ-C4 has the effects as the following:

It enhances the effect of anticancer drugs;

It can promote B cell mitosis;

It can promote the recovery of radiation-damaged hematopoietic system;

It has a promoting effect on phagocytes;

It has the function of protecting the thymus to increase immunity and protecting the bone marrow to produce blood.

D. The toxicity test

XZ-C4 can be taken for a long time. Acute toxicity experiments have shown that the LD50 cannot be made and is a safe prescription. It has been used in this specialist clinic for many years. Some patients have been taking it for 3 to 5 years, or even 8 to 10 years, to protect the body's immunity, to prevent cancer recurrence and metastasis. This prescription can be taken orally for a long time and is quite a safe anti-cancer and anti-metastasis oral medicine.

(5) The following series preparations of XZ-C immune regulation and control anti-cancer Chinese medicine have many experimental and clinical contents and are long in length. Therefore, only the names are listed here, and the introduction is omitted.

1. XZ-C5 Liver Cancer Powder

2. XZ-C6 Bangyu Cancer Powder

3. XZ-C7 Lung Cancer Powder

4. XZ-C8 Husui Shengxue Powder, attenuated by radiotherapy and chemotherapy

5. XZ-C9 pancreatic cancer, prostate cancer powder

6. XZ-C10 Brain Tumor Powder

The above-mentioned scientific research Chinese medicinal preparations for anti-cancer, anti-metastasis, and recurrence of various cancers have been applied to clinical oncology clinics for 30 years on the basis of experimental research, and have achieved good results.

Our oncology specialist outpatient clinic deals with scientific research Chinese medicine preparations for various complications of cancer:

1. Anticancer Xiaoshui Decoction-Indications of pleural fluid and ascites

2. Shugan Jianghuang Decoction-Indications of liver cirrhosis and jaundice

3. Postoperative Aikang San-Helping recovery after radical cancer surgery

4. Hunger soup-for cancer patients with poor appetite

5. Tongyou Decoction-for postoperative anastomosing stenosis

6. Nianlian Songjie Decoction-for patients with adhesions after cancer

The preparations of the above-mentioned scientific research pilot products have been observed by a large number of patients in the wood tumor specialist outpatient department for many years, and they have achieved good results, alleviating the suffering of patients, improving the quality of life, and prolonging the survival period.

Summary table of main pharmacological effects of XZ-C immune regulation and control anti-cancer Chinese herbal medicine (anti-cancer promotion)

	Increased white blood cells	Enhanced phagocytosis	Enhance cellular immune	Enhance humoral immune	Enhanced hematopoietic function	Improve gastrointestinal function		Enhance the weight of the thymus	Promote bone marrow cell proliferation	Enhanced T cell function	Enhanced NK cell activity	Enhanced LAK cell activity	Enhanced IL-2 activity levels	Enhance the level of interferon IFN activity	Enhanced TNF activity levels	Enhanced CSF colony stimulating factor	Antagonistic WCBYC ↓	Inhibition of platelet coagulation and antithrombosis		Antitumor	Anti-metastasis	Antiviral	Anti-cirrhosis	Liver protection	Eliminate free radicals	Protein synthesis	Anti-HIV	
Z-C-A-APL																				+	+							
Z-C-B-SLT																				+	+							
Z-C-C-SNL																				+	+							
Z-C-D-PGS	+	+	+	+	+	+	6	+	+	+	+		+	+	+	+	+		9	+	+	+			+	+		20
Z-C-E-PCW		+	+				2	+	+				+	+	+	+	+		7	+	+	+						12
Z-C-F-AMK		+	+	+	+	+	5			+			+				+		3	+		+		+				11
Z-C-G-GUF		+	+	+		+	4				+		+					+	3	+		+		+		+		11
Z-C-H-RGL	+		+		+		3		+	+			+	+		+			5	+					+			10
Z-C-I-PLP	+	+	+	+	+	+	6		+	+								+	3	+		+					+	12
Z-C-J-ASD	+	+	+	+	+		5	+	+	+			+	+	+		+	+	8	+				+				15
Z-C-K LWF		+	+				2									+		+	2	+	+							5
Z-C-L-AMB	+	+	+	+	+		5	+	+	+	+	+	+	+					7	+		+				+		5
Z-C-M LLA	+	+	+	+			4	+		+									2	+						+		5
Z-C-N-CZR		+					1								+			+	2	+	+							5
Z-C-O-PMT	+	+	+	+	+	+	6	+	+	+						+			4	+		+	+	+	+	+		16
Z-C-P-STG							0												0	+								1
Z-C-Q-LBP	+	+	+	+	+		5		+	+	+	+	+		+	+	+		8	+	+				4			16
Z-C-R-NSR		+					1	+		+								+	3	+	+		+	+				8
Z-C-S-GLK	+	+	+	+	+		5			+		+	+	+	+		+		6	+	+			+		+	+	16
Z-C-T-EDM	+	+	+	+	+		5	+		+			+	+		+	+		6	+		+			+			14
Z-C-U-PUF		+	+	+			3			+	+	+							3	+				+				8
Z-C-V-ABB							1		+	+	+			+					4	+								6
Z-C-W-SCB	+						1		+									+	2	+				+	+			5
Z-C-X-SDS							0				+	+	+						3	+								4
Z-C-Y-PAR							0				+	+	+		+	+			5	+								6
Z-C-Z-CVQ							0							+					1	+								2

The research of the new concepts and new methods for cancer metastasis treatment(1)

A. *The series products of XZ-C immune regulation and control anti-cancer and anti-metastasis Chinese medicine developed exclusively by XUZE.*

Aims or Goals:

It is to find and screen anti-cancer and anti-metastatic Chinese herbal medicines from Chinese medicines

The purposes:

It is to screen out "smart anticancer drugs" that are non-drug resistant, highly selective, non-toxic and side effects, and can be taken orally for a long time.

The Route:

From experimental research to clinical verification, applied to clinical practice on the basis of successful animal experiments.

The method:

To this end, we conducted animal experimental studies on 200 Chinese herbal medicines believed to have anti-cancer effects in traditional Chinese medicine to screen new anti-cancer and anti-metastatic drugs.

Our laboratory has carried out the following experimental research on the cancer suppression rate of Chinese herbal medicine

↓

(1) Our laboratory adopts the method of in vitro culturing of cancer cells, and has carried out the screening experiment for anticancer rate of Chinese herbal medication	*(2) Our laboratory used EAC or S180 or H22 cancer cells to be inoculated to create cancer-bearing animal models, and to conduct a screening test of the anti-tumor rate of Chinese herbal medicine in cancer-bearing animals.*

↓

In vitro tumor inhibition screening test:	*In vivo tumor suppression screening test*
Culture cancer cells in vitro to observe the direct damage of drugs to cancer cells	*Making animal models:*
	The mice inoculated with EAC or S180 or H22 cancer cells
↓	↓
In-test tube screening test:	
Put crude drug products (500ug/ml) into the test tube for culturing cancer cells to observe the inhibitory effect on cancer cells.	**The experiment groupings are as the followings:**
	In each batch of experiments, 240 mice were divided into 8 groups, each with 30 mice, the 7th group was the blank control group, and the 8th group used 5-FU or CTX as the control group.
↓	
200 kinds of Chinese herbal medicines considered by traditional Chinese medicine to have anti-cancer effects, one by one in vitro screening test	↓
↓	*After 24 hours of inoculation, each mouse was fed with a certain amount of crude pharmaceutical powder, and the long-term feeding was used to observe the survival period, toxicity and side effects, calculate the prolonged survival rate, and calculate the tumor inhibition rate.*
Test and compare the control with fiber cell culture under the same conditions	
↓	↓
The experimental results are :	**The experimental results:**
48 species have good tumor inhibition rate, and the other 152 species (Chinese herbal medicines traditionally believed to have anticancer effects) have no obvious tumor inhibition effects.	*48 kinds of Chinese herbal medicines do have a certain tumor inhibition rate. Among them, 26 have good anti-tumor effects.*
↓	↓
It was further create cancer-bearing animal models for in vivo tumor inhibition rate screening test.	*The 48 kinds of traditional Chinese medicines with good tumor inhibition rate were selected from this screening, and then optimized combination.*

	↓
	Repeated tumor inhibition rate experiments and immune experiments in cancer-bearing animal models
	↓
	Finally, a preparation of XUZEChina1-10 (XZ-C1-10), a traditional Chinese medicine for immune regulation and anti-cancer with Chinese characteristics, was developed.

B. The immune function of XZ-C immune regulation and control anti-cancer Chinese medication on the molecular level

There are mainly six aspects for XZ-C immune regulation and control anti-cancer Chinese medicine, summarized as the following:

(1) The effective ingredients of XZ-C Chinese herbal medicine can protect the immune organs and increase the weight of the thymus and spleen.	(2) The active ingredients of XZ-C immunoregulatory anti-cancer Chinese medicine have effects on the proliferation, differentiation and hematopoietic function of bone marrow cells	(3) XZ-C immunomodulatory anti-cancer Chinese medicine has the effect of enhancing T-dimensional cell immunity	(4) XZ-C immune regulation anti-cancer Chinese medicine enhances the activity of NK cells. In the body's immune surveillance function, NK cells are the first line of defense against tumors	(5) The active ingredients of XZ-C immunomodulatory anti-cancer Chinese medicine have an effect on interleukin-2 (IL-2)	(6) XZ-C immune regulation and anti-cancer Chinese medicine has the effect of inducing and promoting the induction of interferon among the active ingredients

(1) The effective ingredients of XZ-C Chinese herbal medicine can protect the immune organs and increase the weight of the thymus and spleen:

XZ-C-7 (ASD)	XZ-C-O(PMT)	XZ-C-W(SCB)	XZ-C-M(LL)	XZ-C-L
Is used on the mouse 15g/kgX7d ↓ Increased weight of thymus and spleen	Is used on the mouse 6g/kgX 7d ↓ Increased weight of thymus and spleen	Is used on the mouse SCB liquid 7d ↓ Increased weight of thymus and spleen	Gavage LLA liquid for mice 7d ↓ Increased weight of thymus and spleen	↓ Increased weight of thymus and spleen

↓

(2) **The active ingredients of XZ-C immunoregulatory anti-cancer Chinese medicine have effects on the proliferation, differentiation and hematopoietic function of bone marrow cells**

XZ-C-D (PMT)	XZ-C-Q (LBP)	XZ-C-D (TSPG)	XZ-C-E (PEW)
PMT 50mg// (kg-d) X 3d On the 9th day, mouse bone marrow hematopoietic stem cell proliferation (CFU-S) increased significantly	LBP10mg/(kg.d)X3d killed on the 9th day, mice (CFU-S) increased significantly	Panax ginseng is an effective ingredient that promotes hematopoietic function and stimulates the proliferation of bone marrow hematopoietic cells. TSPG can induce hematopoietic growth factors	The effective part can enhance the production of colony stimulating factor (CSF) and increase WBC in mice.

↓

(3) XZ-C immunomodulatory anti-cancer Chinese medicine has the effect of enhancing T-dimensional cell immunity

XZ-C-L (LBP)	XZ-C4 has the function of regulating the
LBP can obviously promote the proliferation of T cells and increase the lymphocyte transformation of tumor patients.	immune system and can activate T cells in the lymph node to stimulate the secretion of hematopoietic growth factors in the erythrocytes

↓

(4) XZ-C immune regulation anti-cancer Chinese medicine enhances the activity of NK cells. In the body's immune surveillance function, NK cells are the first line of defense against tumors

XZ-C (SDS)	XZ-C-G (GL)	XZ-C-L (AMB)
Promote the activation of NK cells by IL-Z	0.5mg GL ip can enhance NK cell activity in the liver	Both 0.5g/kg and lg/kg can significantly enhance mouse NK cell activity

↓

(5) The active ingredients of XZ-C immunomodulatory anti-cancer Chinese medicine have an effect on interleukin-2 (IL-2)

XZ-C (EBM)	XZ-C-Y (PEP)
EBM polysaccharide can significantly enhance the production of human IL-2 at 100ug/ml	PEP polysaccharide has strong immune activity and can promote the production of IL-2

↓

(6) XZ-C immune regulation and anti-cancer Chinese medicine has the effect of inducing and promoting the induction of interferon among the active ingredients.

IFN has a broad-spectrum anti-tumor effect and immunomodulatory effect. IFN can inhibit tumor cell proliferation and activate NK cells to kill tumor cells.

XZ-C-Z	XZ-C-E	XZ-C-D
VCQ polysaccharide 250mg/ kg, can significantly increase the level of IFN-y produced by mouse spleen cells	There is immune regulation by methyl tuckahoe polysaccharide. Promote INF, indirect antiviral	Ginseng triol soap (PTGS) Can induce human whole blood cells, mononuclear cells produce IFN-a, IFN-v

↓

C. Biological response modifiers (BRN) and BRM-like Chinese medicines and tumor treatment

BRM has created a new field of tumor biotherapy. At present, as the fourth program of tumor treatment, BRM has received extensive attention from the medical community.

$\downarrow$

What is BRM?

Oldhain founded the biological response modifier (BRM) or BRM theory in 1982. On this basis, the family proposed the fourth modality of cancer treatment, a biological treatment.

$\downarrow$

According to BRM theory:

Under normal circumstances, there is a dynamic balance between the tumor and the body's defenses. The occurrence and metastasis of tumors are completely caused by this dynamic balance.

If the already imbalanced state is artificially adjusted to a normal level, It can control the growth of the tumor and make it disappear.

$\downarrow$

Our exclusive research and development products:

The research of XZ-C immunoregulation and anti-cancer Chinese medicine's mechanism of action suggests that:

Cancer invasion and metastasis are determined by the ratio of two factors:

a. The biological characteristics of tumor cells
b. The host's influence on its constraints

Cancer can be controlled if the two factors keep the balance; Imbalance between the two factors makes cancer progress

$\downarrow$

We take the path of modernization of traditional Chinese medicine, promote the integration of traditional Chinese and Western medicine at the molecular level, and integrate with the modernization of international medicine.

The mechanism of XZ-C immune regulation and anti-cancer Chinese medicine is similar to that of BRM medicine:

Biological response modifiers include the following anti-cancer mechanisms:

<u>The BRM roles are as the followings</u>:

1. *Promote the enhancement or reduction of the effect of the host's defense mechanism on the immune suppression of the tumor-bearing host to achieve the ability of immune response to the tumor.*

2. *Administer natural or genetically recombined biologically active substances to enhance the host's defense mechanism.*

3. *Modified tumor cells to induce a strong host response.*

4. *Promote the differentiation and maturation of tumor cells and make them normalized into cells.*

5. *Reduce the side effects of cancer chemotherapy and radiotherapy, and enhance the tolerance of the host.*

The main pharmacological effect of XZ-C immune regulation and control anti-cancer Chinese medicine is anti-cancer and promotion of immune function, and its anti-cancer mechanism is:

XZ-C type BRM functions are as the following:

1. *Activate the body's immune cell system; Promote the enhancement of the effect of the host's defense mechanism and achieve the ability of immune response to cancer.*

2. *Activate the immune cytokine system of the body's anti-cancer mechanism; improve immune surveillance.*

3. *Protect Thymus and Increase immune function ; protect bone marrow function which produce blood.*

4. *Reduce the side effects of radiotherapy and chemotherapy.*

5. *It can make the thymus gland enlarge and gain weight, and make the thymus gland not progressively shrink. Improve the body's immunity and immune surveillance.*

As mentioned above, the mechanism of action of XZ-C anti-regulatory anti-cancer Chinese medicine is basically similar to that of BRM, and the same therapeutic effect can be obtained in clinical use.

↓

Therefore, XZ-C immunomodulatory anticancer Chinese medicine has BRM-like effects and curative effects.

↓

Combine the current advanced molecular oncology theory with ancient Chinese herbal medicine resources at the molecular level of Chinese and Western medicine, and use the BRM theory as a bridge to integrate with the international advanced theory and practice of modern molecular tumors.

XZ-C1
(Smart Anti-cancer)

Pharmacodynamics:	Pharmacology:	Toxicology:
96%-100% inhibits cancer cells and has no effect on normal cells.	It strengthens the body, eliminates the evil without hurting the body, has a strong inhibition on cancer cells, but does not inhibit normal cells.	Acute toxicity experiments have shown that there is no obvious side effect, and the LD50 is difficult to make. It is a fairly safe prescription.

XZ-C4
(Thymus Protector and Increase Immune function Ai Kang San)

Pharmacodynamics:	Pharmacology:	Toxicology:
Anti-tumor effect on H22 mice bearing liver cancer: The tumor inhibition rate of XZ-C4 in the second week was 55% The tumor inhibition rate of XZ-C4 in the 4th week was 68% The pain inhibition rate of XZC4 in the 6th week was 70%	_Promote lymphocyte transformation, enhance cellular immune function, increase white blood cells, inhibit cancer cells, protect the immune organs, protect the thymus from atrophy, and protect the Thymus._	XZ-C4 can be taken for a long time. Acute toxicity experiments show that the LD50 cannot be produced. It is a safe prescription. Some patients take it for 3-5 years, or even 8-10 years, to maintain the body's immunity. Prevent cancer recurrence and metastasis. This prescription can be taken orally for a long time and is quite safe and effective anti-cancer and anti-metastasis oral medicine.

It is to strive to take the innovative path of anti-cancer metastasis with Chinese characteristics!

It is to take the path of modernization of traditional Chinese medicine, promote the combination of traditional Chinese and Western medicine at the molecular level, and integrate with international medicine modernization.

**The study of new concepts and new methods for cancer metastasis treatment (2)**

A. The clinical validation

XZ-C immunomodulatory Chinese medicine has become the basis for experimental research and applied in clinical practice

It was to perform clinical verification on the basis of successful animal experiments.

Establish an oncology clinic
Establish an anti-metastatic and recurrence scientific research team

Keep outpatient medical records
Establish a regular follow-up observation system
Observe the long-term effect

↓

Observed on a large number of patients for 3-5 years
Even clinical observation for 8-10 years

↓

Have long-term follow-up and evaluable data

↓

The standard of efficacy is:

Good quality of life and long life span

XZ-C immunomodulatory Chinese medicine preparations have achieved remarkable curative effect after 12 years of application to a large number of patients with cancer of the Middle East.

↓

Adopt XZ-C immune regulation to target cancer cells on the way of metastasis, improve immune surveillance, and open up the third area of anti-cancer metastasis therapy.

↓

It can improve the quality of life of patients with advanced cancer, enhance immunity, improve immunity and control ability, increase the body's anti-cancer ability, increase appetite, strengthen physical strength, protect bone marrow, and enhance hematopoietic function.

↓

Patients who have taken the drug for a longer period of time have very few recurrences after surgery, and the rate of metastasis is very small. Most of the patients who have metastasized and relapsed can be stabilized without further metastasis. Many patients with metastases of multiple organs in the body have also stable medical condition, and they control metastasis, can significantly prolong survival.

B. <u>The clinical application verification data</u>

<u>The clinical information:</u>

From 1994 to November 2002, XZ-C immunomodulatory anti-cancer Chinese medicine was used to treat 4698 cases of stage Ill, IV or metastatic or recurrent cancer, including 3051 males and 1647 females. The oldest was 86 years old and the youngest was 11 years old. Histopathological diagnosis or B-ultrasound, CT, MR imaging diagnosis, according to the International Anti-Cancer Alliance staging standards, all cases are patients above stage III.

The treatment results are as the followings:

The symptoms are improved, the quality of life is improved, and the survival period is prolonged.

After taking XZ-C immunoregulatory Chinese medicine, 4277 patients with intermediate and advanced cancer who were re-diagnosed for more than 3 months all had different degrees of symptom improvement after taking the medicine, with an effective rate of 93.2%. See Table 1 for general information. See Table 2 for the improvement of the quality of life of patients, see Table 3 for changes in external application of swelling, and Table 4 for pain relief.

Table 1

General data of 4277 cases of recurrence and metastasis

		Liver cancer	Lung cancer	Stomach cancer	Esophagus cancer	Rectal anal cancer	Colon cancer	Breast cancer	Pancreatic cancer
Number of Case		1021	752	668	624	328	442	368	74
Male:Female		4:1	4.4:1	2.25:1	3.1:1	1:1	2.1:1	All of Female	3.2:1
Location of lesions Or Cancer foci	Primary	694 (68.8%)	699 (93.9%)						
	Metastasis	327 (31.2 %)	53 (6.1%)						
Common transfer sites in this group		Lung metastasis (2%) , from stomach 27.2% Xili (19.5%) comes from the rectum 12%, (a few,	Supraclavicular lymph node metastasis (11,6%) Brain metastasis ((3.1%) Bone metastasis ((4.6%)	Metastasis to the liver (23.8%) Metastasis to the lung (3%) Peritoneal metastasis (29.1%) Supraclavicular metastasis (6.1%)		Recurrence rate (14.8%) Metastatic liver (7.0%)	Metastatic liver (16.0%) Peritoneal metastasis (6.0%) Bone metastasis (5.0%)	Supraclavicular lymph node metastasis (17.5%) Axillary lymph node metastasis (15.0%)	Metastatic liver (11.7%) Retroperitoneal metastasis (39.1%)
Age	Peak ages	30-39 (76.2)	50-69 (71.6)	40-69(73.4)		40-49(75.2)	30-69 (88.0)	40-59 (65.9)	40-59 (70.0)
	Youngest	11	20	17		27	27	29	34
	Oldest	86	80	77		78	76	80	68

Table 2

Observation of curative effect of 4277 cases to improve the quality of life of patients with advanced cancer

	Spirits	Appetite	Body strength increase	Generally conditions get better	Weight gain	Sleep better	Improving ability of moving, limited activities alleviated	Walk as usual,Live indepent	For light work
Get better	4071	3986	2450	479	2938	1005	1038	3220	479
%	95.7	93.2	57.3	11.2	68.7	23.5	24.3	75.3	11.2

Table 3

The changes of 56 cases of metastatic nodules after external application of XZ-C ointment
The swollen supraclavicular lymph nodes in the neck

	disappear	Reduce 1/2	Turn soft	No change
Number of cases	12	22	14	8
%	21.4	39.2	25.0	14.2
Total effective rate (%)	85.7			

Table 4

Pain relief after oral administration of XZ-C medicine and external application
of XZ-C anticancer pain relief ointment in 298 patients

Clinical manifestations	Mild relief	Pain		
		Significantly reduced(1/2)	Disappear	Invalid
Number of cases	52	139	93	14
(%)	17.3	46.8	31.2	4.7
Total effective rate (%)		95.3		

→

In improving the quality of life (according to the Karnofsky score standard)
The average score is 50 points before taking the medicine, 80 points after three months of treatment, and some reach 90 or 100 points.

→

The survival analysis is as the following:

The patients from outpatients are difficult to compare due to different stages and severity of illnesses.

The patients in this group are all at stage III or above, with metastasis and dysfunction of different tissues and organs. According to previous statistics, the median survival time of such patients is about 6 months. The longest cases in this group have reached 14 years, and the average survival time of the remaining cases is more than 1 year.

→

a. 1 case of liver cancer recurrence and resection after long-term use of XZ-C drug for 14 years;

b. Another case of liver cancer took xz-c drug for 10 and half years;

c. 3 cases of lung cancer could not be cut after open chest, long-term use of XZ-C medicine has been 3 and half years;

d. 2 cases of remnant gastric cancer took XZ-C medicine for 8 years;

e. 3 cases of rectal cancer recurrence after surgery have taken XZ-C medicine for 3 years;

f. 1 case of breast cancer metastasis to liver and ribs has been taking XZ-C medicine for 8 years;

g. One case of renal cancer recurrence after surgery has been taking XZ-C medicine for 9 and half years.

These patients have undergone long-term outpatient review, taking medicines, and taking medicines, and their condition is controlled in a stable state. The long-term growth period with tumors has significantly extended the survival period.

The analysis of prolonged survival is as the following:

1. The typical cases who cannot be operated, radioed or chemotherapy, only take XZ-C immunoregulatory anti-cancer Chinese medicine for more than 5 years are:

(1) Di xx left upper left lung central lung cancer with left lung metastasis, served XZ-C1+4+7 for 5 years.

(2) Huang xx esophageal cancer has been taking medicine for 5 years.

(3) Huang X x middle esophageal cancer has been taking medicine for 5 years.

(4) Huang xx primary massive liver cancer has been taking XZ-C medicine for 5 years.

(5) Qi xx primary liver swallow has been taking XZ-C medicine for 5 years. (See medical records for details)

The analysis of prolonged survival is as the following:

2. *The typical cases of using XZ-C immunomodulatory traditional Chinese medicine for 4 years are as follows:*

(1) After becoming xx with abdominal distension, the tumor cannot be removed by exploratory surgery and has been taking XZ-C medicine for 4 years..

2) It has been taken XZ-C medicine for 7 years since pancreatic adenocarcinoma detection can not remove cancer lesions.

(3) Li xx's primary massive liver cancer could not be removed by Tongji Hospital while exploration. He has been taking XZ-C medicine for 4 years.

(4) Ke xx's primary liver cancer could not be removed by 301 Hospital, while exploration and he had been taking XZ-C medicine for 5 years. (See medical records for details)

(10). Immunopharmacology of XZ-C
immunomodulation anti-Chinese medication

1). Compared with immunopharmacology of western medicine, traditional Chinese medicine has its own characteristics and advantages.

2). Through long-term clinical experience, Chinese medicine has accumulated *a large number of prescriptions that have the effect of regulating the body's immune function, especially tonic Chinese medicines generally have the effect of regulating immune vitality*.

3). Both single-medicine and prescriptions of traditional Chinese medicine will have multiple active ingredients, unlike western medicine (synthetic medicine) which is a single-structure substance.

4). *The role of traditional Chinese medicine is multifaceted. In addition to regulating the immune function, it also has a certain effect on the overall functional system*.

5). The main role of XZ-C Chinese medicine immunomodulators is to *regulate cellular immunity (Cellular immunity)* to regulate various immune cell-mediated immune responses, including cytokines or lymphokines.

6). *The immune regulation function of traditional Chinese medicine mainly acts on stem cell immunity, such as thymus, gonads and lymphatic system, T, B cells and various cytokines*.

7). *Ancient Chinese medicine has the notion that righteous qi is not weak and evil qi does not enter, which constitutes a part of the theory of Chinese medicine.*

8). *Its essence is to maintain overall functional balance and enhance disease resistance. Its main function is to enhance the immune function of the body.*

9). *In fact, tonic drugs are based on immunopharmacology.*

10). *Immunopharmacology is an emerging edge discipline that serves as a bridge between pharmacology and immunology. The traditional Chinese medicine of XZ-C immunomodulator has obvious immune promoting effect.*

11). **Clinical application observation and adaptation range of Anti-tumor Metastasis and Recurrence of XZ-C Immunomodulation Chinese Medicine XZ-C1-10**

1)). The various distant metastatic cancers:

Such as liver metastasis, lung metastasis, bone metastasis, brain metastasis, abdominal lymph node metastasis, mediastinal lymph node metastasis, cancerous pleural effusion, cancerous ascites, can come to Wuchang Shuguang Oncology Specialist Clinic to apply XZ-C immune regulation to resist metastasis treatment,

Follow the steps of metastasis to intervene and block cancer cells during metastasis to prolong life.

2)). After completing the course of various radiotherapy and chemotherapy, you should continue to come to the clinic to take XZ-C1+4 immunoregulatory Chinese medicine to consolidate the long-term curative effect and prevent recurrence.

3)). In the course of radiotherapy and chemotherapy, if the reaction is serious and cannot continue, they can come to Shuguang Tumor Patent No. 1 Clinic and continue to use XZ-C immunomodulation therapy to prevent metastasis and recurrence.

4)). In advanced age or frail patients with other diseases who cannot receive radiotherapy or chemotherapy, they can come to Shuguang Oncology Specialty Clinic and use XZ-C immune regulation to treat metastasis and recurrence.

5)). If you can't find it through surgical exploration, you can come to Shuguang Cancer Specialist Clinic XZ-C immunomodulation treatment.

6)). After palliative surgery, you can come to Shuguang Oncology Specialty Clinic for XZ-C immunomodulation anti-metastasis therapy.

(11) <u>The theoretical system of XZ-C treatment is formed</u>

The book "New Concepts and New Methods of Cancer Treatment" published that Professor Xu Ze spent 20 years on his own and worked hard to complete the basic and clinical research of the National Science and Technology Commission's "Eighth Five-Year Plan" research topics.

Bin Wu, Lily Xu

Nearly a hundred scientific research papers summarized by a series of scientific research results were published in the form of new books.

In this book the theoretical system of XZ-C cancer treatment formed by us is the theoretical basis and experimental basis for cancer treatment and has been undergoing clinical observation and verification. It can be summarized as the following diagram:

During XZ-C laboratory animal experiment it was found:

a. *Removal of the thymus can create a cancer-bearing animal model.*
b. *As the cancer progresses, the thymus gland gradually shrinks*

↓

The discovery of the cause:

atrophy of thymus, weakened immune function

↓

The theoretical basis of treatment was to put forward:

XZ-C immune regulation and control------protection of Thymus and increase immune function

---

↓

The exclusively developed product:

XZ-C immune regulation preparation 1-10

↓

The clinical verification:

Over the past 16 years, more than 12,000 patients with advanced cancer have been observed and followed up in the outpatient clinic, which can improve the quality of life and prolong the survival period, and the curative effect is satisfactory.

Diagram : XZ-C Theoretical System of Cancer Treatment

2

This book preliminarily proposes a new concept of XZ-C cancer treatment on cancer therapy and analyzes and compares it with traditional therapies. It is analyzed with the following table:

Table The comparison between XZ-C new concept of cancer therapy and Traditional Chemotherapy Cancer Therapy

	XZ-C new concept of cancer therapy	Traditional Chemotherapy Cancer Therapy
Theoretical basis	New concept thinks: **Healing or cure should be through regulation and control rather than killing**	Traditional conception: The goal of treatment must be to kill cancer cells
Cause and mechanism:	1. Thymus atrophy 2. Immune function is weak	Not yet
The theoretical basis and experimental basis of treatment	1. Immune regulation and control 2. Protection of Thymus and increasing of immune functions	Not yet
Treatment principles	Establish a comprehensive treatment view	1. Single target to kill cancer cells 2. One-sided view of treatment

Treatment mode	**Full treatment:** Surgery + Biology Immune regulation **Short-term treatment:** Chemotherapy and radiotherapy No long range Not excessive	Radiotherapy + chemotherapy Or Chemical + radiotherapy Or radiotherapy + chemotherapy on simultaneous step
Treating medication	XZ-C immunomodulatory preparation 1-10 1. Modernization of Chinese medicine; 2. Combining Chinese and Western medicine at molecular level	Cytotoxic drugs (killing both cancer cells and normal proliferating cells)
Complications, side effects	no	1. Toxic side effects, 2. some have serious side effects, **3. and some even have immune function failure**, 4.radiotherapy damage is permanent
Curative effect	Improve survival quality and prolong survival	Remission for a few months, it may relapse and progress
Medical expenses or costs	Greatly reduced medical expenses	High medical expenses my country is nearly 100 billion yuan a year
The Prospect	Try to walk out a new path to overcome cancer	The effect is 5%, still lingering

3

The exclusive scientific research products have been developed

1). The series products of XZ-C immune regulation and control anti-cancer Chinese medicine (introduction)

2). The research on XZ-C immune regulation and control anti-cancer Chinese medicine (Introduction)

Secret level: Grade A (A)

The research on XZ-C Immunomodulation Anti-cancer Chinese Medicine:

Table of Contents

1. Overview

2. The experimental research and clinical verification work that has been carried out

3. Immunopharmacology of XZ-C Immunomodulation Chinese Medicine

4. Pharmacodynamics research of XZ-C immunomodulatory anti-cancer Chinese medicine

5. The cytokine research induced by XZ-C4 anti-cancer traditional Chinese medicine

6. Toxicology research of XZ-C immune regulation anti-cancer traditional Chinese medicine

7. About the effective ingredients of XZ-C immune regulation anti-cancer Chinese medicine

8. The principles of XZ-C prescriptions

9. About the immune function effect of XZ-C drug immunomodulation and anti-cancer Chinese medicine at the molecular level

10. About the anti-tumor components of XZ-C drug immune regulation and control anti-cancer Chinese medicine: structural formula, location, anti-tumor effect

11. The source background and completion process of the subject (tortuous process)

12. How can we get out of the boudoir

4

A large number of clinical cases have been verified XZ-C immune regulation and control anti-cancer Chinese medication

1). List of cancer cases and some typical cases treated

Shuguang Oncology Specialist Outpatient Department

March 8, 2011

2). Anti-cancer, anti-cancer metastasis research, scientific and technological innovation, scientific research results series:

XZ-C immune control anti-cancer Chinese medicine for cancer treatment

Table of Contents

1. *List of some cases of liver cancer treated by XZ-C immunoregulatory anti-cancer Chinese medicine*
   (Case 1-----Case 189)

2. *List of some cases of pancreatic cancer treated by XZ-C immune regulation anti-cancer Chinese medicine*
   (Case 190----Case 218)

3. *List of some cases of XZ-C immunoregulatory anti-cancer Chinese medicine in the treatment of gastric cancer*
   (Case 219------Case 288)

4. *List of some cases of lung cancer treated by XZ-C immunoregulatory anti-cancer Chinese medicine*
   (Case 289-----Case 358)

5. *List of some cases of esophageal cancer treated by XZ-C immunoregulatory anti-cancer Chinese medicine*
   (Case 359-------Case 446)

6. *List of some cases of breast cancer treated by XZ-C immunoregulatory anti-cancer Chinese medicine*
   (Case 447--------Case 481)

7. *List of some cases of colorectal cancer treated by XZ-C immunoregulatory anti-cancer Chinese medicine*
   (Case 482------Case 649)

8. *List of some cases of XZ-C immunomodulatory anti-cancer Chinese medicine for treatment of cholangiocarcinoma*
   (Case 650------Case 679)

3). **Anti-cancer, anti-cancer metastasis research, scientific and technological innovation, scientific research results series**

Some typical cases of XZ-C immune regulation and control anti-cancer Chinese medicine for treatment of malignant tumors

Table of Contents

1. *Treat some typical cases of liver cancer*

2. *Some typical cases of postoperative adjuvant treatment of pancreatic cancer*

3. *Some typical cases of adjuvant treatment after gastric cancer*

4. *Some typical cases of postoperative adjuvant treatment of lung cancer*

5. *Some typical cases of postoperative adjuvant treatment of esophageal cancer*

6. *Some typical cases of adjuvant treatment after breast cancer surgery*

7. *Some typical cases of postoperative adjuvant treatment of <u>colorectal cancer</u>*

8. *Some typical cases of adjuvant treatment after <u>gallbladder cancer</u>*

9. *Some typical cases of postoperative adjuvant treatment <u>of kidney cancer and bladder cancer</u>*

10. *Some typical cases of postoperative adjuvant treatment such as <u>thyroid cancer and retroperitoneal tumors</u>*

11. *Some typical cases of <u>non-Hodgkin's lymphoma</u> treatment*

12. *A typical case of chemotherapy + XZ-C Chinese medicine in the treatment of <u>acute lymphoblastic leukemia</u>*

13. *Some typical cases of <u>ovarian cancer and cervical cancer</u> treatment*

5

What are the reforms in the book? What are the innovations?

The third monograph "New Concepts and New Methods of Cancer Therapy" is an innovative concept and content, which has both experimental research basis and clinically verified "New Concepts of Cancer Therapy".

1). *The following is the reform and innovation of traditional therapy proposed by XZ-C internationally or nationally.*

(1) Now the whole world is a single cancer cell killing, which is a one-sided treatment. <u>XU proposes to reform into a comprehensive treatment.</u>

(2) Now that the whole world is dominated by radiotherapy and chemotherapy, <u>the XU initiative should be reformed into surgery + immune regulation as the main, and radiotherapy and chemotherapy as supplementary.</u>

(3) Now that the whole world is systemic intravenous chemotherapy for solid tumors, <u>XU proposes to reform into target organ intravascular chemotherapy.</u>

(4) Now chemotherapeutics are non-selective and should be researched and innovated as selective intelligent anti-cancer drugs. XZ-C1-4 have the selective for the cancer and the normal cells.

(5) <u>Now that chemotherapy has not been tested for drug sensitivity, XU suggested that drug sensitivity test should be conducted (to avoid blindness).</u>

(6) At present, all tumor specimens have not been cultured for cancer cells. <u>XU suggested that all tumor specimens should be cultured for cancer cells (individualized and selective).</u>

(7) The design of radical surgery should be further studied and perfected. XU pointed out that the current radical operation is flawed; several metastasis approaches only pay attention to the solution of lymphatic metastasis;**there are also blood circulation and planting**, which are not paid attention to.

XU proposed that surgical design and technology should be reformed, and tumor-free technology should be emphasized to prevent the blood spread of cancer cells during surgery.

(8) Now postoperative chemotherapy is mostly carried out in the chemotherapy department, and the chemotherapy doctors and nurses do not understand the conditions seen during the operation.

XU proposes that postoperative chemotherapy should be postoperative adjuvant chemotherapy or perioperative adjuvant chemotherapy should be reformed to be carried out by surgeons and nurses, because postoperative drug pump administration, observation, and follow-up surgeons can master the whole treatment process.

(9) For half a century, traditional therapies believe that radiotherapy and chemotherapy are based on killing cancer cells.

This book proposes that healing should be through regulation and control rather than killing.

2). The following arguments in this book are the first to be proposed in the world, all of which are original papers, leading the world:

(1) The first international proposal:

Thymus atrophy and weakened immune function are the causes and pathogenesis of cancer.

This is an internationally leading achievement of independent intellectual property rights, and it is the first time that it has been proposed internationally after a novelty search.

(2) The first international proposal:

XZ-C immunomodulation therapy---Thymus protection and increasing immunity, is the theoretical basis and experimental basis for cancer treatment.

(3) The first international initiative:

The goal or target of cancer treatment must be aimed at both the tumor and the host at the same time, and a comprehensive treatment view must be established.

The one-sided treatment view of simply killing cancer cells should be overcome or the unilateral treatment view of simply killing cancer cells should be overcome.

(4). The first international initiative:

The model of multidisciplinary organic integration is mainly long-term treatment: Surgery + biological therapy + immunotherapy;

Short-term treatment is supplemented:

Radiotherapy and chemotherapy, which should not be long-term or excessive.

(5) The first in the world to point out:

The Questions and four comments on the problems and disadvantages of systemic intravenous chemotherapy for solid tumors.

(6) The first international proposal:

It is recommended that systemic intravenous chemotherapy for abdominal solid tumors should be reformed into target organ intravascular chemotherapy.

(7) The first international proposal:

There are three main manifestations of cancer in the human body. The third form is cancer cells that are on the way to metastasis.

(8) The first international proposal:

The "two points and one line" theory of the whole process of cancer development. Cancer treatment should pay attention to two points, and should pay more attention to cut off the first line.

(9) The first international proposal:

Three steps of anti-cancer metastasis treatment, three strategies are proposed.

(10). The first international proposal:

Open up the third area(blood circulation) of anti-cancer treatment.

3). The following arguments in this book are first proposed nationwide:

(1) It was to do the animal experiments in our experimental surgery laboratory, which the experimental research was to explore the cause, pathogenesis, and pathophysiology of cancer.

Since 1985, the results and scale have been the first in the country.

(2) The excision of the thymus to create animal models, and to use cancer-bearing animal models to conduct in vitro and in vivo anti-tumor experiments with traditional Chinese medicines.

Among 200 traditional Chinese medicines, 48 Chinese medicines of XZ-C were screened out through in vivo experiments on tumor-bearing animal models, which are all internationally advanced.

(3) It has been 40 years to keep medical records of specialist outpatient clinics, with more than 12,000 cases, follow-up, follow-up for the long-term, and to establish the cancer clinic medical records database.

(4) XZ-C immunomodulatory Chinese medication $_{1-10}$ exclusively developed has been clinically verified for 18 years, and has achieved the good results after the long-term observation and follow-up.

4). XZ-C has proposed the following reform and development proposals for traditional therapy:

In the last two centuries, there have been two leaps in the treatment of malignant tumors

↓

The first time it was in 1890 that Haisted proposed the concept of very curative tumors.

↓

The second time was Fish integrated chemotherapy into radical surgery (adjuvant chemotherapy or neoadjuvant chemotherapy) in the 1970s

↓

Since then, the treatment of malignant tumors has been stagnant, and the death of malignant bell tumor is still the first

↓

The radical mastectomy →

Extended radical mastectomy or super radical mastectomy →

Modified radical mastectomy →

Chemotherapy is integrated into radical surgery (adjuvant chemotherapy or neoadjuvant chemotherapy) →

Radiation and chemotherapy target to kill cancer cells, while killing proliferating cells and immune cells →

Failed to improve the efficacy, and toxic and side effects occurred, reducing immunity →

Professor Xu Ze has reformed and develop and initiative the following 6 points:

Professor Xu Ze puts forward the following 4 suggestions for reform and development:

It is proposed that the design of radical resection needs further research and improvement	Proposed that tumor-free technology in tumor surgery is extremely important	Prevent cancer cell blood implantation during surgery	During the operation, it is necessary to prevent shedding cancer cells from planting	Point out that the cure should be through regulation, not just killing	A comprehensive treatment view should be established for both the host and cancer cells	Point out that chemotherapy needs to be further researched and improved	Questioned the administration route of systemic intravenous chemotherapy for solid tumors	Advocate the reform of systemic intravenous chemotherapy for solid tumors into target organ intravascular chemotherapy	Advocate the reform of adjuvant chemotherapy after cancer surgery to spinal vein catheter pump chemotherapy

5). The following original papers are first published in this book:

1) One of the etiology and pathogenesis of cancer may be thymic atrophy and weakened immune function (Chapter 2).

2) The theoretical basis and experimental basis of the therapeutic principles of XZ-C immune regulation and control therapy for Thymus protection and immune function promotion (Chapter 3).

3) The target of cancer treatment must be aimed at both the tumor and the host at the same time to establish a comprehensive treatment view (Chapter 5).

4) It is to propose a comprehensive treatment plan (Chapter 6).

The full-course treatment:

The surgery therapy is the main focus, and it is to add the biological treatments, and immunomodulation therapy.

The short-term treatment:

The radiotherapy and chemotherapy are the mainstays, but it is not excessive.

5) Analysis and questioning of the administration route of systemic intravenous chemotherapy for solid tumors (Chapter 11).

6) The proposal that systemic intravenous chemotherapy for solid tumors should be reformed into target organ intravascular chemotherapy (Chapter 12).

These six original papers proposed a series of reforms and innovations on traditional chemotherapy and chemotherapy.

7) It was to excision of the thymus to create animal models, and to use cancer-bearing animal models to conduct in vitro and in vivo anti-tumor experiments with traditional Chinese medicines.

Among 200 traditional Chinese medicines, 48 traditional Chinese medicines of XZ-C were screened out through in vivo experiments on tumor-bearing animal models, and XZ-C1-10 Immune regulation and control anti-cancer Chinese medicine preparation were developed.

8) XZ-C immunomodulatory anti-cancer Chinese medicine research overview, experimental research and clinical efficacy observation (Chapters 26 and 27).

9) Strategic thinking and suggestions for conquering cancer.

The above nine original scientific research papers may enable cancer treatment to embark on a new path to overcome cancer, and to a new era of immune-modulated targeted therapy.

This is not the end of subject research, but the beginning of a new path <u>to translational medicine</u> <u>through the development of translational medicine.</u>

<u>Translational medicine</u> has developed rapidly internationally in recent years. This new medical research model advocates patient-centeredness, discovers problems and proposes problems in clinical work, conducts in-depth basic research, and then quickly transfers the results of basic research to clinical application to improve the overall level of medical care and ultimately enable patients Benefit. The XZ-C series of scientific research results are fully in line with this new medical research model.

The research focus of translational medicine in my country, <u>the modernization and internationalization of Chinese medicine and traditional Chinese medicine is</u> one of the key contents of translational medicine research in my country.

There have been several years after the publication of this monograph and new book, <u>we will start to organize the transformation and development of XZ-C scientific research results.</u>

Science-is the endless frontier.

Our scientific research work has always followed the scientific development concept, based on known science, facing the future of medicine, and looking forward. After 60 years of hard work, facing the frontier of science, we strive for innovation and progress.

- *To conquer cancer, we must come from the clinic, go through experimental research, and go to the clinic to solve the actual problems of patients;*
- *We must seek truth from facts, speak with facts and data; we must constantly surpass ourselves and advance ourselves;*

- *In scientific research, we should emancipate the shackles of the mind, get rid of traditional old concepts, and base ourselves on independent innovation and original innovation;*
- *Our 60-year scientific research route is to discover problems to ask or to raise problems to research problems to solve problems or explain problems.*

This is how the road has come, step by step, and with difficulties.

Under the guidance of the scientific development concept, we hope to embark on an innovative path of anti-cancer and metastasis with Chinese characteristics and independent intellectual property rights.

- *Our medical oncology research model is patient-centered, discovering and asking questions from clinical work, conducting in-depth basic research on animal experiments, and then turning the results of basic research into clinical applications to improve the overall level of medical care and ultimately benefit patients.*

- *Experimental surgery is extremely important in the development of medicine, which is a key to open the forbidden area of medicine.*

The prevention and treatment of many diseases has been applied in clinical practice and promoted the development of medical undertakings after many animal experimental studies and stable results have been obtained.

6

Research Theoretical Innovation Content of new concepts and new methods of cancer metastasis treatment

This book carefully analyzes and summarizes our 60 years of clinical treatment experience in tumor surgery and more than 30 years of laboratory research results, formed a new understanding and new concept of cancer metastasis with its own characteristics and new technologies and new methods for cancer anti-metastasis therapy.

Its main contents include:

1. *Three manifestations of cancer in the human body;*

2. *"Two points and one line" theory of the whole process of cancer development;*

3. *The "eight steps and three stages" theory of cancer metastasis;*

4. *The third area of human anti-cancer metastasis therapy;*

5. *The "three steps" of metastasis treatment,*

6. *And the self-developed ZX-C (XU ZE-CHINA) immune regulation and anti-cancer series of traditional Chinese medicine preparations.*

The following new understandings, new theories, and new concepts *have not been* mentioned in the literature or in textbooks so far.

All of them are the theories, which our knowledge has risen to, that is, the experience and lessons of <u>clinical practice</u> after half a century from the author himself,, and more than 30 years of <u>experimental research, analysis, reflection, and understanding</u>.

They are all independent intellectual property rights of independent innovation and original innovation.

1. Theoretical innovation content

(introduction)

The following is our exclusive theoretical system of the new concept of cancer anti-metastatic treatment, which is the independent and intellectual property rights of independent innovation and original innovation.

(1) *We first discovered and proposed a new theory or new theoretical understanding in the world:*

It is proposed that there are three manifestations of cancer in the human body. The third form of the manifestation of cancer in the human body is the group of cancer cells that are in the process of metastasis or on the way of metastasis.

Our new concept of cancer metastasis treatment believes:

There are three manifestations of cancer in the human body:

1. *The first manifestation is primary cancer*

2. *The second manifestation is metastatic cancer*

3. *The third manifestation is a group of cancer cells on the way to metastasis*

The first two manifestations may be visible, tangible, or visible through endoscopy, or visible through imaging.

The third manifestation is cancer cells that are in the process of metastasis. They are invisible or intangible and cannot be detected by endoscopy, B-ultrasound, CT, MRI, etc. These potential, hidden, and erratic cells are metastasizing.

The millions of metastatic cancer cell populations on the way are the greatest enemy in the lives of threatening cancer patients.

The goal or "target" of cancer treatment should be for the three forms of cancer that exist in the human body, namely:

1. ***One of the goals of functional therapy, targeting the primary lesion:***

2. ***The second goal of treatment is to target metastatic cancer;***

3. ***The third goal of treatment is to target the cancer paper cell population on the way to metastasis.***

If this new theory or new theoretical understanding is confirmed and accepted, it may cause a series of changes and updates in the diagnosis and treatment of chain reaction-like tumors:

(1) Changes and updates on the concept of cancer <u>treatment</u>;

(2) Changes and updates in the understanding of cancer <u>treatment goals or "targets"</u>;

(3) Changes and updates on cancer <u>diagnosis methods</u>;

(4) It will surely cause major changes and updates in the <u>research and development of anti-cancer and anti-metastasis drugs</u>;

(5) It is bound to cause major changes and updates <u>to cancer treatment models and methods</u>;

(6) <u>The research on cancer metastasis and recurrence will surely lead to a revolution and update from the cell-level oncology of cytopathological morphology to the molecular-level oncology of molecular biology and gene expression</u>.

Why should it be proposed that the third manifestation of cancer in the human body is the metastasis of cancer cells, cancer cell groups, and micro-cancer thrombi that are in the process of multi-step and multi-factor metastasis?

This problem has not been recognized by people so far, and it has not attracted enough attention, let alone the methods and countermeasures of how to diagnose and treat cancer cells in metastasis, in another word, there is no specific discussion on the methods and countermeasures of how to diagnose and treat cancer cell populations during metastasis.

This is because this third form of existence has not been mentioned in the literature and textbooks, has not yet been recognized, and has not yet been paid attention to.

In fact, the key to anti-cancer metastasis is to encircle, block or interfere with cancer cells in the process of metastasis, and to cut off the new treatment mode.

To conquer cancer, we should update our thinking and change our concepts, and cancer treatment should have a comprehensive therapeutic concept

The main manifestations of cancer in the human body, two different concepts of cancer treatment, there are two different understandings:

(1) *Xu Ze (XU ZE) new concept of cancer treatment believes that there are three forms, and there are three manifestations of cancer in the human body:*

The first manifestation is the primary cancer;

The second manifestation-metastatic cancer;

The third manifestation is the metastasis of cancer cells, cancer cell groups and micro-cancer thrombi that are in the process of metastasis.

The goal or "target" of treatment is also for these three manifestations:

One is for the first manifestation-primary cancer;

The second is for the second manifestation-metastatic cancer;

The third is to target the third manifestation-the cancer cell population on the way to metastasis.

This new concept believes that cancer is manifested in three forms in the human body, which is relatively complete and comprehensive. It clarifies the dynamic relationship, causality and subordination between the three, and is a complete new concept of cancer therapy.

It fully explains the whole process of cancer development and how to control the whole process of cancer cell metastasis.

This new theory will bring the dawn of victory over cancer.

2) The traditional concept of cancer therapy believes that there are two manifestations:

The first manifestation----primary cancer;

The second manifestation------metastatic cancer.

Traditional cancer therapeutic goals or "targets" are sufficient for these two forms:

One is for the first manifestation-primary cancer;

The second is for the second manifestation-metastatic cancer.

This traditional therapeutic concept has been used for more than one hundred years, and its treatment goals or "targets" are for these two manifestations-primary cancer or metastatic cancer. It is to treat these two "targets" in isolation, while the dynamic relationship, causality, and affiliation between the two are not considered. That is, how the primary cancer is formed into metastatic cancer and how to stop its metastasis is not covered.

Therefore, the traditional concept of cancer therapy believes that there are only two manifestations of cancer in the human body, which this understanding is not comprehensive, incomplete and defective.

Therefore, the treatment implemented based on this understanding is only aimed at these two. There are two forms---------primary cancer foci and metastatic cancer foci, while ignoring cancer cells on the way to metastasis.

As we all know, metastasis is the biological characteristics and biological behavior of malignant tumors. The difference between benign tumors and malignant tumors is that the former does not metastasize while the latter metastasizes.

Anti-metastasis is the key to cancer treatment.

Without blocking the cancer cells that are in the process of metastasis, the metastasis of cancer cells cannot be controlled, and therefore, it is difficult to obtain the possibility of full cancer treatment.

(2) **Xu Ze (XU ZE) first proposed another new theory or new theoretical understanding in the world:**

It is the "two points and one line" theory of the whole process of cancer development.

In fact, *the treatment of cancer should not only pay attention to two points, but also pay attention to the first line.* <u>*Cutting the first line is the key to fighting cancer metastasis*</u>

However, it is believed that in the treatment of cancer, only two points have been recognized and valued at home and abroad in the past and present, and the first line has been ignored. The cancer treatment strategies should be changed.

What is two points and one line?

The two points are the starting point of metastasis, the primary cancer; and the end of metastasis, the metastatic cancer.

The first line is a route between the primary cancer foci and the metastatic cancer foci where cancer cells travel a long distance to metastasize to distant organs.(see Figure 1)

Primary cancer   Invasion and metastasis route   Metastatic cancer

$$A \xrightarrow{\hspace{4cm}} B \hspace{3cm} C$$

Figure1. Two-point and one-line schematic diagram of the whole process of cancer metastasis

Note: A: Primary cancer, starting point of metastasis;
            B: The route of the invasion and transfer process;
            C: Metastatic cancer, the end of metastasis.

Regardless of the starting point of the primary tumor or the end point of metastasis, when the cancer has grown to a certain size, it will become a new source of exfoliated cancer cells.

This metastatic cancer can be transferred again and become the starting point for the second round of metastasis. Such transfer can continue to develop slowly and eventually endanger the patient's life. (See Figure 2)

$$A \hspace{2cm} B \hspace{2cm} C(A') \hspace{2cm} B' \hspace{2cm} C'$$

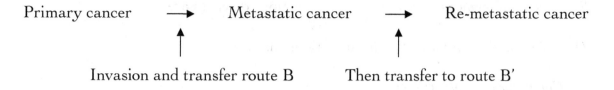

Figure 2 Diagram showing the re-metastasis of metastatic cancer

Note: A′ is the new starting point;
         B is the re-transfer route;
C′   is the new end point.

Traditional cancer treatment often only pays attention to "two points", but ignores the "first line".

__XU ZE's new concept of cancer treatment believes that not only should pay attention to "two points", but also cut off the front line.__

Through the experimental data of the laboratory to explore the law of metastasis and the analysis of the clinical data of a large number of metastatic cases in the Cancer Specialty Clinic of the Anti-Cancer Metastasis and Recurrence Laboratory, we have concluded that the metastasis process of cancer cells is quite similar to that of infectious diseases:

1.   The three major elements of infectious diseases are:

(1) There is a source of infection;

(2) The route of infection;

(3) People who are susceptible.

The metastasis of cancer cells also includes:

(1) **Source of metastasis;**

(2) **Route of metastasis;**

(3) **Organs and tissues that are easy to implant.**

2.   The countermeasures to deal with infectious diseases are

(1) Isolate and treat patients with infectious diseases;

(2) *Cut off the route of infection*;

(3) Strengthen the immunity of susceptible people.

XU ZE believes that similar principles can also be used to deal with cancer metastasis:

(1) **Treatment of primary cancer;**

(2) **Cut off the way of metastasis to prevent and kill cancer cells in the process of metastasis;**

(3) **Enhance the body's immune surveillance ability and improve the anti-cancer power of the patient's body.**

However, the control of infectious diseases (such as the control of SARS) is an epidemiological control *in the macro environment of society*, and the control of cancer cell metastasis is only an intervention in the *host's internal visceral microenvironment.*

The above processing schemes are summarized in Figure 3.

Infectious disease	Expand in the macro environment of society	(1)Isolation treatment, Control the source of infection (2) Cut off the infection route: (3) Enhance immunity of susceptible people.

Cancer metastasis	In the human body microenvironment	Treatment of metastatic source (primary cancer or metastatic cancer) (surgical resection, radiotherapy)
		(2) Cut off the metastasis pathway (immunity, biology, gene, small dose chemotherapy, traditional Chinese medicine BRM)
		Prevent and block and kill cancer cells on the way of metastasis;
		Enhance the body's immune surveillance ability and improve the patient's ability to fight cancer.

Figure 3 Treatment plan for infectious diseases and cancer metastasis

In summary, it can be seen that the new concept of XU ZE cancer treatment not only pays attention to the surgical resection, radiotherapy, and chemotherapy of primary and metastatic tumors, *__but also pays attention to the interception and killing of cancer cells on the way of metastasis__*.

__This new theory, called "two points and one line", has the following important meanings:__

(1) *__More specific and specific on how to resist metastasis target or target.__*

(2) *__To further supplement and improve the countermeasures or strategies of traditional cancer therapy.__*

(3) *__Emphasize that anti-metastasis should not only attach importance to "two points", but also attach importance to "one line".__*

__Only by cutting off cancer cells on the way to metastasis can the therapeutic effect be improved.__

(4) *__It enables people to have a clearer concept of cancer metastasis, a more specific protagonist, and a new theoretical basis, which is helpful for clinicians to rationally__*

design and use their own various treatment methods and explore new treatment method.

(5) *Open up a new field of basic cancer experimental research and clinical practice research.*

(3) Xu Ze (XU ZE) first proposed the "three steps" of anti-cancer metastasis treatment in the world

1. Try to break each transfer step.

First of all, It is to clarify the concept of each transfer step, and to make the "target" of treatment more specific and more clear.

In order to scientifically design the interception of each transfer step, and each break, the concept of each step of the transfer process must be clearer and clearer, and the "target" of each step must be clear before it can be maneuverable so as to study and explore the prevention and control measures for each step.

Considering the design of treatment strategies, after in-depth analysis, I further summarized the "eight steps" of cancer cell metastasis into "three stages".

The first stage is the stage before the cancer cells separate from the mother or primary tumor and enter the blood vessels;

The second stage is the stage where the plaque cells pass through the blood vessel wall and enter the blood circulation;

The third stage is the stage when cancer cells penetrate the blood vessel wall to implant on the target organ tissues and metastases form.

In order to scientifically design the block for each metastasis step, we design and formulate prevention and treatment strategies at each stage based on the "eight steps" and "three stages" on the molecular mechanism of cancer cell metastasis, and call this *XU ZE anti-cancer metastasis therapy "Three Steps".*

2. XU ZE's three major strategies for anti-cancer metastasis (ie three steps)

(1) *The first step in anti-cancer metastasis*

The route of cancer cell metastasis at this stage:

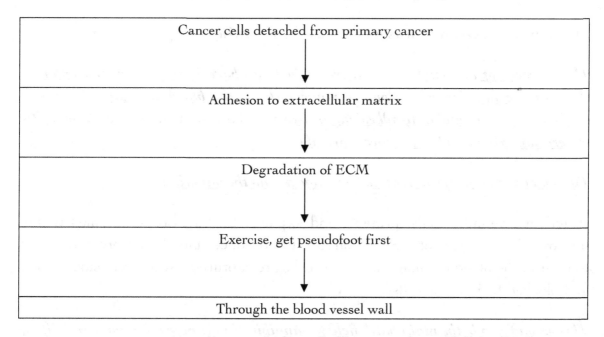

Cancer cells detached from primary cancer

↓

Adhesion to extracellular matrix

↓

Degradation of ECM

↓

Exercise, get pseudofoot first

↓

Through the blood vessel wall

The prevention countermeasures are as the followings:

The treatment "targets" at this stage are mainly <u>anti-adhesion, anti-degradation, anti-movement, and anti-cancer invasion.</u>

The goal of treatment:

It prevents cancer cells from entering the blood vessels and achieves the purpose of "fighting the enemy outside the country".

(2) **The second step of anti-cancer metastasis**

The route of cancer cell metastasis at this stage is as the followings:

From the cancer cells drill through the blood vessel wall into the blood circulation.

Cancer cells are in contact with various immune cells while floating in the blood circulation, and may be captured and swallowed by various immune cells in the bloodstream and cannot survive.

Most of the cancer cells in the circulatory journey are damaged by the circulating immune cells or the strong blood flow impact and shear force. Very few surviving cancer

cells escape the surveillance of the immune cells in the blood circulation and most of them form tiny tumor thrombi, can adhere to microvascular endothelial cells, degrade basement membrane, and penetrate outside the blood vessel.

The prevention countermeasures are as the followings:

The "target" of anti-metastasis therapy in this phase is to protect and enhance the immune function of various immune cells in the blood circulation, activate immune cytokines and anti-adhesion, anti-exercise, anti-platelet aggregation, anti-hypercoagulation, and anti-cancer thrombus.

The goals of cancer Treatment at this stage are as the following:

It activates immune cells, protects and expands the function of thymus tissue, improves immunity, protects the marrow and produces blood, and promotes stool to float in the blood circulation. Cancer cells are captured, swallowed, surrounded and blocked by immune cells.

This second step is the main battlefield for annihilating cancer cells that are drifting in the blood circulation, and is also the main strategy to intervene to prevent the metastasis of cancer cells.

(3) **The third step of anti-cancer metastasis**

The route of cancer cell metastasis at this stage is as the followings:

Cancer cells evade the surveillance of immune cells in the blood circulation and the killing of immune cells, traverse the blood vessel wall, and anchor to settle in the appropriate organs and tissues in the local microenvironment. The tumors form new microvessels and gradually form metastatic cancer foci.

The prevention countermeasures are as the followings:

1, **To improve the local microenvironment and tissue immunity,**

2, **adjust the local microenvironment, make it unfavorable for survival and implantation,**

3, **inhibit angiogenesis factors,**

4, **and inhibit the formation of new blood vessels.**

In summary, XU ZE's anti-cancer metastasis treatment is "three steps". The space for the treatment of cancer metastasis is located in the blood circulation and the time is located in three different stages. It emphasizes on improving host immunity.

It can be summarized as Table 1.

Table 1

XU ZE "Three Steps" of Anti-cancer Metastasis Treatment

Cancer metastasis stage	The route of mestastasis	Prevention countermeasures
Anti-metastatic first step: Pre-circulation stage of cancer cell invasion	Separation of cancer cells from primary cancer ↓ Degradation of ECM ↓ Adhesion and de-adhesion ↓ Movement ↓ Before entering the blood vessel	Anti-adhesion; Anti-degradation; Anti-exercise or movemnt; Anti-matrix metal protease; Keep cancer cells out of blood vessels

Anti-metastatic second step: Cancer cells are transported in the blood circulation stage	Cancer cells groups and microscopic small tumor thrombi were floating in the blood circulation, undergo phagocytosis and capture by immune cells, and are damaged by the impact of blood flow shear force.	Enhances and activates various immune cells and cytokines in the circulation, enhances immune function, and is the main battlefield for annihilating cancer cells on the way to metastasis; Anti-adhesion; Anti-platelet aggregation; Anticancer thrombus
The third step of anti-metastasis: Cancer cells escape the bleeding cycle and anchor the "target" organ tissue stage	After the cancer cells escape the blood vessels, they anchor the "target" organs and tissues to implant, form new blood vessels, and form metastases lesions.	TG; Inhibit angiogenesis factor; Inhibit blood vessel formation; Increase immune regulation; Improve local microenvironmental tissue immunity

Metastasis is not the end point. After the metastasis grows to a certain size, it will separate, invade, and metastasize cancer cells, and become a new source of cancer cell metastasis. At this time, both the primary and metastatic foci can become the source of cancer cell shedding and metastasis, the main way is blood metastasis.

Therefore, the more and larger the metastatic cancer, the more cancer cells enter the blood circulation. The number of immune cells in the blood circulation in the patient's machine is far from enough to control a large number of cancer cells shed from the cancerous foci into the blood circulation.

The body's immune function is seriously unbalanced, or even immune function failure, which can cause blood circulation.

At this time, there is a crisis of immune cell immune function in the patient's body?

There are only two ways, one is foreign aid and the other is endogenous:

1. *The foreign aid is stem cell transplantation;*

2. *The endogenous is biological therapy, immunotherapy, gene therapy, molecular biological therapy, Chinese medicine therapy, XZ-C immunomodulation Chinese medicine therapy, and BRM therapy.*

(4) Xu Ze (xu ZE) first proposed to open up the third field of human anti-cancer metastasis treatment in the world

What is the third field of anti-cancer metastasis therapy?

All targeting the third manifestation of cancer in the human body-the treatment of cancer cells on the way to metastasis, can be called the third area of anti-cancer therapy.

The first manifestation of cancer in the human body is the primary cancer. All treatments for primary cancer (surgical resection or radiotherapy), we call it the first area of cancer treatment;

The second manifestation of cancer in the human body is metastatic cancer. All treatments for metastatic cancer (radiotherapy, chemotherapy, intervention and some local treatment measures) can be called the second area of anti-cancer treatment.

Now we recognize and propose that the third manifestation of cancer in the human body is: cancer cells in the process of metastasis, then, all the treatments and treatment methods for cancer cells in the process of metastasis, let us call it human The third area (or third front) of anti-cancer treatment.

1). The necessity of the third area of anti-cancer treatment is proposed as the following:

Why is there still recurrence and metastasis after standardized radical resection?

Now that a radical resection of the primary cancer and radical regional lymphadenectomy have been done, why are there still recurrences and metastases after a period of time after surgery? Where are the remaining cancer cells lurking after surgery? how many cancer cells are there? What are the rules of its activities?

After repeated thoughts, I realized that these cancer cells may have surpassed the regional lymph nodes before surgery;

Or some cancer cells have entered the bloodstream through the lymphatic tract;

Or some cancer cells were squeezed into the blood circulation during the operation.

All of these cancer cells are in the process of metastasis. They potentially and slowly metastasize. Some are monitored, swallowed, and captured by immune cells in the blood circulation, and some are in a dormant state.

Some quickly formed metastases. However, in some patients, the formation of metastases is very slow, which can take several months, or even 1-2 years, during which the cancer cells on the way of metastasis can be in a static and dormant state.

These cancer cells in the metastasis process are actually the third manifestation in the human body. We must find countermeasures to develop anti-cancer treatment for the third area.

2). The possibility of blocking cancer cells during metastasis

The formation of metastases is the most important turning point in the development of cancer.

Before metastasis, cancer is only a local problem, and local therapy can be used to achieve good results. But at this stage, local therapy can no longer cure patients. **Therefore, we set anti-metastasis therapy as the top priority.**

At this stage, millions of cancer cells enter the blood circulation every day, but less than 0.01% of them can eventually become metastases.

Therefore, preventing or killing these metastatic cancer cells for anti-metastatic treatment is not only necessary but also possible.

If the appropriate measures are taken to activate immune cells in the blood, improve immune surveillance of immune cells, and activate immune cytokines, it will be very possibility and useful to stop the possibility of cancer cells on the way to metastasis.

How is it to stop metastatic cancer cells on the way to metastasis?

Cancer patients usually have a weakened immune function, especially the cellular immune function is declining with the development of tumors.

However, many studies have shown that although tumor-bearing hosts may have systemic immune deficiencies, they generally have normal T cell responses. It can stimulate effective anti-cancer responses in animal experiments and clinical research.

The key is how to break the tumor's suppression of the immune system and stimulate an effective immune response especially based on T cells.

How can it is to effectively regulate the host's immune function?

It is to improve the local immune microenvironment so that it can facilitate the development of the host's anti-cancer effect, which is an important and effective measure to prevent postoperative metastasis and recurrence of cancer and eliminate residual cancer cells. It is an important part of comprehensive cancer treatment.

3). **The circulatory system has a large number of immune surveillance cells**

Cancer cells are chased, intercepted, captured and swallowed by immune cells in the blood circulation. Therefore, it can be said that blood circulation is the main battlefield for annihilating cancer cells on the way to metastasis, and immune cells are the vital force to kill algae cells.

The circulatory system has a large number of immune surveillance cells, which can kill and swallow cancer cells with heterogeneous antigens. Coupled with the impact and shear force of the bloodstream, it is difficult for a single swimming cancer cell to survive.

In order to escape the pursuit of immune cells, cancer cells will adhere to the platelets and adheres to the inner wall of the blood vessel. The endothelial cells in the inner wall of the blood vessel make amoebic movement, pass through the capillaries and settle in new organs, gradually forming new metastases.

4). **XU ZE specific plan for anti-cancer metastasis treatment**

According to the biological behavior of modern oncology of cancer metastasis and the theory of recurrence and metastasis, our laboratory has been looking for new anti-metastatic drugs from natural medicines in Chinese medicine for several years.

In experimental studies in tumor-bearing animals, we use traditional Chinese medicine and a combination of Chinese and Western medicine to interfere with all aspects of the metastasis step, chase and intercept. It was also developed the XZ-C immune control series of anti-metastasis programs and measures, such as :

1. Z-C-TG anti-angiogenesis;

2. Z-C-AS Tumor Dissolving Plug;

3. Z-C-MD is resistant to invading and puncturing blood vessels;

4. Z-C-LM antigenicity,

5. Z-C-Ind anti-PGE2;

6. VA and Z-C-CA calcium channel blockers resist invasion;

7. Z-C-GB anti-adhesion;

8. Z-C-TIMP is resistant to drug resistance;

9. vXZ-Cl only inhibits cancer cells, we do not kill normal cells;

10. XZ-C4 chest protector promotion;

11. XZ-C8 marrow protects blood;

12. Brucea javanica enters human lymph nodes.

__The comprehensive measures of the above treatment programs have achieved good results in the outpatient clinical practice of our anti-cancer collaboration group.__

__Cancer metastasis is a complex process with multiple steps and multiple links. The treatment of cancer metastasis should be a comprehensive approach in many aspects and cooperate with each other. It cannot be pinned on one medicine and one method.__

We have scientifically designed and adopted different treatment plans and countermeasures for the transfer steps. See Table 2 as the following. It is to achieve the same goal of anti-metastasis for the transfer step.

Table 2. Xu ZE new concept anti-cancer metastasis treatment new model (The treatment plan and countermeasures implemented for cancer metastasis steps)

Transfer steps	Treatment strategy	XZ-C immune regulation Chinese medicine and its effect
Primary cancer proliferation	Surgery, radiotherapy, chemotherapy	XZ-C1 inhibits cancer cells XZ-C4 chest protector XZ-C8 marrow protects blood
Tumor angiogenesis	Inhibit angiogenesis	Z-C-TG anti-angiogenesis Z-C-CA anti-adhesion
Invasion of basement membrane	Anti-adhesion, anti-motion Inhibit hydrolase activity	XZ-C-K (LWF) anti-adhesion Ind anti-PGE2 2-C-MD anti-exercise
Penetration into blood vessels or lymphatic vessels	Anti-adhesion, anti-motion Inhibit hydrolase activity	2-C-MD anti-invasive blood vessel 2-C-K (LWF)
In the blood of the circulatory system	Anti-platelet aggregation and anticoagulation, Biological response regulation BRM	XZ-C1+4 immune regulation Z-C-K (LWF) anti-adhesion 2-C-N (CZR) anti-platelet aggregation Z-C-LM XZ-C-ASP cancer thrombus
Formation of tumor thrombus	Promoting blood circulation	XZ-C1+4 immune regulation 2-C-K (NSP) Anti-cancer thrombus 2-C-N (CZR)
Piercing out the vessels	Anti-adhesion, anti-exercise, anti-hydrolytic protease activity	Z-C-MD anti-invasion of blood vessels
Formation of metastases	Surgery, radiotherapy, chemotherapy	XZ-C1+4 immune regulation Z-C-TG inhibits blood vessel growth
Metastatic lymph node	Fat-soluble agents	Brucea javanica emulsion lipid carrier Into the lymph nodes

(5) XU ZE's new concept and model for cancer treatment

1. *It is to strengthen immunotherapy and improve the side effects of chemotherapy*

(1) The side effects of traditional chemotherapy:

In cancer chemotherapy, immune function is often suppressed, bone marrow hematopoietic function is suppressed, WBC and PLT decrease, liver and kidney function damage, gastrointestinal function damage, nausea, vomiting, abdominal distension, anorexia and other toxic and side effects, as shown in Figure 4.

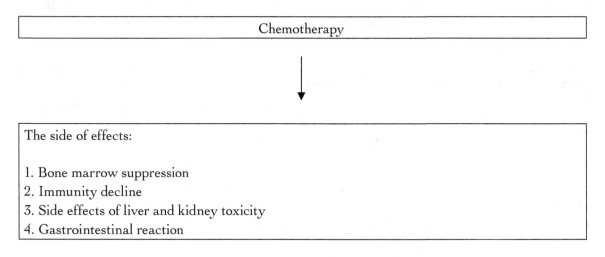

Figure 4 Side effects of traditional chemotherapy

(2) **The countermeasures against the new concept of XU ZE:**

The way to improve the toxicity of chemotherapy is to strengthen supportive therapy and adopt effective measures to protect the host.

With immune regulation Chinese medicine, XZ-C4 protects thymus and improves immunity; Use XZ-C8 to protect bone marrow hematopoietic function and produce more stem cells;

Use XZ-C immunomodulatory drugs to enhance the strength of those who squeeze.

The figure 5 is as the following:

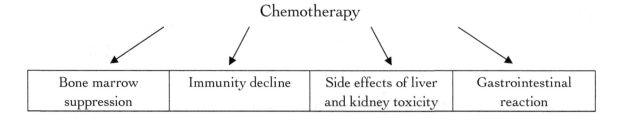

↑

> 1. XZ-C Immunomodulation Chinese Medicine Treatment
> 2. Chinese medicine treatment
> 3. BRM treatment
> 4. Immunobiological therapy

Figure 5. The methods of anti-toxic side effects of chemotherapy

2. **It is to change intermittent treatment to continuous treatment**

(1). **Xu Ze's new concept and new model of cancer treatment are continuous treatment**

In the intermittent period, XZ-C1+4 immunomodulatory Chinese medicine therapy or BRM therapy is used.

The XZ-C1 immunomodulatory drug has been screened after 7 years of tumor-bearing animal experiments and has undergone 10 years of clinical verification.

It only inhibits swallow cells, has no effect on normal cells, and can invigorate the spleen and stomach.

XZ-C4 can protect the thymus, prevent its atrophy, increase immunity, and prevent immune decline.

To get treatment during the intermittent period, the continued use of XZ-C anti-cancer Chinese medicine can not only control the proliferation of cancer cells, but also protect the function of immune organs such as the thymus.

The comprehensive application of chemotherapeutics and XZ-C immune regulation Chinese medicine can not only reduce the toxicity of chemotherapy, but also enhance and consolidate the efficacy of chemotherapy to prevent the loss of immune monitoring, as shown in Figure 6 as the following.

The occurrence and development of tumors are determined by the comparison between the host's immune function and the biological characteristics of the tumor itself. Cancer invasion and metastasis are also determined by two factors, that is, the biological characteristics of tumor cells and the host's influence on the constraints are compared. If the two are balanced, they will be controlled, and if the two are out of balance, they will progress.

Traditional radiotherapy and chemotherapy both promote the decline of immune function, which will make the two more unbalanced. The new model of XU ZE cancer treatment is to find ways to improve the immunity of patients, promote the rise of immunity to balance, make it beneficial to curb the development of tumors and strengthen immune monitoring.

chemotherapy		chemotherapy		chemotherapy		chemotherapy
↓	Intermittent peroid	↓	Intermittent peroid	↓	Intermittent peroid	↓
↑	Z-Cl+4 immune regulation and control medications	↑	Z-Cl+4 immune regulation and control medications	↑	Z-Cl+4 immune regulation and control medications	↑

Figure 6. The continuous treatment during the intermittent peroid

(2). Traditional intravenous chemotherapy is an intermittent treatment, that is, after 3-5 days of chemotherapy, it takes 3-4 weeks, especially after WBC and PLT return to normal, the second course of chemotherapy can be used. Between these 2 courses During the intermittent period, chemotherapeutics cannot be continued, but during this intermittent period, cancer cells continue to continue cell proliferation and division, which multiplies geometrically. Moreover, due to the suppression of immune function during chemotherapy, during the intermittent period between the two courses of treatment, because cancer cells lose (or reduce) immune monitoring, cell proliferation and division are faster, that is, the longer the course of chemotherapy, the combination The more the medication and the greater the dose, the more severe the immune system will be hit, resulting in loss of immune monitoring, and even recurrence and metastasis during chemotherapy. The tumor shrinks first and then continues to grow (Figure 7).

Such cases are not uncommon. What should we do? We believe that during the intermittent period of the two courses of treatment, immunotherapy should be continued in the following mode:

Chemotherapy		Chemotherapy		Chemotherapy
Decrease of immunity and Lose Monitor cancer cell division due to decreased immunity and lose control of cancer cell division		Decrease of immunity and Lose Monitor cancer cell division due to decreased immunity and lose control of cancer cell division		Decrease of immunity and Lose Monitor cancer cell division due to decreased immunity and lose control of cancer cell division
Bone marrow suppression Immunity decline Side effects of liver and kidney toxicity Gastrointestinal reaction		Bone marrow suppression Immunity decline Side effects of liver and kidney toxicity Gastrointestinal reaction		Bone marrow suppression Immunity decline Side effects of liver and kidney toxicity Gastrointestinal reaction

Figure 7. The cancer can return or relapse during the intermittient period due to no treatment

7

Briefly describe the scientific research process of anti-cancer research

A. Briefly describe the scientific research process

1. Brief introduction of the scientific research process of anti-cancer research

In 1985, Dr. Xu Ze research team sent letters and visits to more than 3,000 patients who had undergone radical resection of chest and general surgery.

The outcome was or It was turn out:

Most patients have recurrence and metastasis within 2-3 years after surgery, and some even occur within a few months after surgery. It made me realize that the operation was successful and the long-term effect was not satisfactory.

The postoperative recurrence and metastasis are the key factors affecting the long-term effect of the operation.

Therefore, a question is also raised :

Studying the prevention and treatment of postoperative recurrence and metastasis is the key to improving postoperative survival.

Therefore, basic clinical research must be carried out. Without breakthroughs in basic research, it is difficult to improve clinical efficacy. So we established the Experimental Surgery Research Institute, and spent 60 years in the following three aspects to conduct a series of experimental research and clinical verification work, which it took a series of experimental studies and clinical verifications in the following three aspects:

(1). It is to explore the mechanism of cancer incidence, invasion and recurrence and metastasis, and find experimental research on effective measures to regulate invasion, recurrence and metastasis.

We have been doing experimental tumor research in our laboratory for 4 years. The topic selection of research projects is to raise questions from the clinic, and attempts to explain some clinical problems through experimental research or solve some clinical problems are all clinical basic research.

(2) The experimental research on finding new anti-cancer, anti-metastasis and anti-relapse drugs from natural medicine and Chinese herbal medicine was done.

The existing anti-cancer drugs kill both cancer cells and normal cells, and have great toxic side effects. Our laboratory has passed the tumor suppression test in cancer-bearing mice to find new drugs that only inhibit cancer cells without affecting normal cells from natural medicines.. Our laboratory has spent 3 years to conduct anti-tumor screening experiments in cancer-bearing animals on 200 kinds of Chinese herbal medicines commonly used in traditional anti-cancer prescriptions and anti-cancer prescriptions reported in various places.

The result was as the followings:

48 kinds of traditional Chinese medicines with good tumor inhibition rate were screened out, and at the same time, they have good promotion and immune function, and found the traditional Chinese medicine TG which can inhibit the neovascularization.

(3) The clinical verification work is as the following:

Through the above 4 years of basic experimental research to explore the mechanism of recurrence and metastasis, and 3 years of experimental research on screening substances from natural medicines and Chinese herbal medicines, a batch of XZ-C_{1-10} anti-cancer immune regulation Chinese medicines were found. *In the clinical verification of many cases of metastatic cancer patients in late or postoperative period, the application of XZ-C immunoregulatory Chinese medicine has achieved good results, improved the quality of life, improved symptoms, and significantly extended the survival period.*

Recently, we have reviewed, analyzed, reflected on, and experienced clinical practice cases in the past 60 years, as well as the results and findings of more than ten years of cancer-bearing animal experimental research, from the experiment to the clinical, and from the clinical to the experiment, the experimental research and the clinical verification data.

In summary, some of 18 monographs have been published are as the following:

1. <<Conquer cancer and launch the total attack to cancer>> in 2018 by Authorhouse In presses in Bloomington, IN in USA

2. <<Walked out of the new road to conquer cancer>> Volume II in 2019 by Authorhouse in presses in Bloomington, IN in USA

3. <<Walked out of the new road to conquer cancer>> Volume III in 2019 by Authorhouse in presses in Bloomington, IN in USA

4. <<The research on anticancer traditional chinese medication with immune regulation and control>> Volume IV in 2019 by Authorhouse in presses in Bloomington, IN in USA

5. <<Innovation on clinical application theory of cancer prevention and treatment research in the 21st century>> Volume V in 2019 by Authorhouse in presses in Bloomington, IN in USA

6. << Build up the multidisciplinary and the science city of the research base with related to cancer research for conquering cancer>> Volume VI in 2019 by Authorhouse in presses in Bloomington, IN in USA

7. << Create the researvh institute of the environmental protection>> Volume VII in 2019 by Authorhouse in presses in Bloomington, IN in USA

8. << Create an environmental protection and cancer prevention research institute and carry out cancer prevention system engineering>> Volume VIII in 2019 by Authorhouse in presses in Bloomington, IN in USA

9. <<New concepts and new way of treatment of cancer metastasis>> in 2016 by Authorhouse in presses in Bloomington, IN in USA

10. <<The new progress in cancer treatment>> in 2018 by Authorhouse in presses in Bloomington, IN in USA

11. <<New concept and new way of treatment of cancer>> in 2013 by Authorhouse in presses in Bloomington, IN in USA

12. <<The road to overcome cancer >> in 2016 by Authorhouse in presses in Bloomington, IN in USA

13. <<On innovation of treatment of cancer>> in 2015 by Authorhouse in presses in Bloomington, IN in USA

14. << Condense Visdom and conquer cancer>> Volume I in 2018 by Authorhouse in presses in Bloomington, IN in USA

15. <<Condense Visdom and conquer cancer>> Volume II in 2018 by Authorhouse in presses in Bloomington, IN in USA

2. **The ideological understanding and scientific research thinking of our scientific research journey**

Summary

Our 60 years of cancer research work and scientific research journey of thinking and scientific thinking can be divided into three stages. The Introduction in brief is as the followings:

(1) The first stage from 1985 to 1999: **it was the stage which was to find the questions for the cancer treatment and reasons as the following.**

- *It is to find problems from the follow-up results → ask questions → research questions;*

- From the review, analysis, reflection, and discovery of current problems in traditional cancer treatments, it was found that the further research and improvement are needed;

- It was recognized that there is a problem, it should change thinking and change concept;

- It was to sum up the data, collate, collect and publish the first monograph "New Understanding and New Model of Cancer Treatment" in Chinese version published in January 2001 in China.

(B) The second stage after 2001----- *it was the stage that cancer treatment and research was focused on anti-metastasis stage.*

- It was to position or locate the research goal and the "target" of *cancer treatment on anti-metastasis*, and point out that the key to cancer treatment is *anti-metastasis*;

- **It was to conduct a series of anti-cancer metastasis and recurrence experimental research and clinical basis and clinical verification research, and upgrade it to theoretical innovation, and propose the new ideas and new methods for anti-metastasis;**

- It was to summarize the data, compile, organize, and published the second monograph (New Concepts and New Methods of Cancer Metastasis Therapy" published in Chinese version in 2006, and received the award from People's Republic of China News in 2007 for "Three Hundreds, Original Book Award"

(C) The third stage after 2006------ it was the stage for the research of the prevention and treatment of cancer therapy

- It was to conduct *research on the prevention and treatment of the entire process of cancer occurrence and development*

- It was to tightly integrate clinical practice, and propose reforms and innovations, scientific research and development *in response to the current problems and disadvantages of traditional clinical therapies*;

- It was r*ecognizing that the strategy of cancer prevention and treatment must move forward, the way out for cancer treatment is in the "three early time ", and the way out for anti-cancer is prevention;*

- <u>**We have been engaged in oncological surgery for 60 years. There are more and more patients, the incidence of cancer is also rising, and the mortality rate remains high. We deeply understand that cancer must not only pay attention to treatment, but also pay attention to prevention, in order to stop it at the source.**</u>

- It has conducted a series of related studies, summarized information, sorted out, compiled, and published the third monograph "New Concepts and New Methods of Cancer Treatment" published in Chinese version in 2011 in China, later it was translated into English by Dr. Bin Wu, an American medical scholar fellow. The English version was published in Washington on March 26, 2013 and distributed internationally.

B. Thoughts and understanding of our scientific research journey and scientific research thinking

The ideological understanding and scientific thinking of my scientific research journey can be divided into 3 stages. The introduction of these three stages is as the followings:

1. *The first stage*

(1985-1999)

The new discoveries and new understandings

It starts with <u>discovering the existing problems</u>→ <u>ask the questions</u>→ <u>creative or innovative thinking and changing ideas.</u>

In 1985, it was to conduct the letters and visits to more than 3,000 postoperative patients with chest and abdomen cancer that Dr. Xu Ze had done.

It was found that most of the patients recurred or metastasized within 2-3 years after surgery; it was found that **the postoperative recurrence and metastasis are key factors that affect the long-term effect of surgery.**

It is necessary to conduct basic clinical research to prevent cancer recurrence and metastasis. Without breakthroughs in basic research, it is difficult to improve clinical efficacy.

Since experimental surgery is the key to opening the restricted area of medicine, we established a tumor animal laboratory, established an experimental surgery laboratory, and carried out a series of experimental tumor research:

- Carried out cancer cell transplantation;
- Established a cancer animal model;
- Explored the mechanism and law of cancer invasion, metastasis and recurrence;
- Looked for effective measures to regulate cancer invasion, recurrence and metastasis.

The New Discoveries

The things were discovered from experimental tumor researches:

1. *Removal of the thymus can create a cancer-bearing animal model. The research findings: the occurrence and development of cancer have a certain or positive relationship with the host's thymus.*

2. *When our laboratory studies the relationship between cancer metastasis and immunity, the experimental results suggest that metastasis is related to immunity.*

3. *Experimental studies have found that as the cancer progresses, the host's Thymus show progressive atrophy.*

For further research, the Experimental Surgery Institute of Hubei University of Traditional Chinese Medicine was established in March 1991 on the basis of the Experimental Surgery Laboratory. **Professor Xu Ze is the director, and Academician Qiu Fazu is the consultant. The goal and task of his research is to tackle cancer as the main attack direction.**

Since 1994, we have established an oncology specialist outpatient department. Through the review of clinical medical practice cases, the analysis, evaluation and reflection of postoperative adjuvant chemotherapy, we found that there are problems:

① *Adjuvant chemotherapy in some patients failed to prevent recurrence*

② *In some patients, postoperative adjuvant chemotherapy failed to prevent metastasis*

③ *Chemotherapy in some patients promoted immune failure*

From the analysis and reflection of clinical practice cases, the questions were asked : why does the postoperative chemotherapy fail to prevent recurrence and metastasis?

From analyzing and reflecting on the effects of the **chemotherapeutics on the cycle of cancer cells**, *analyzing and reflecting on chemotherapeutic* **drugs inhibiting immunity**, *analyzing and reflecting on the* **resistance of chemotherapeutics**, *and* **then it was to discover that there are problems:**

① *There are still some important misunderstandings in current chemotherapy*

② *There are still several main contradictions in current chemotherapy, which need to be further studied and improved*

It was found from the follow-up results:

The postoperative recurrence and metastasis are the key to the long-term effect of surgery.

So it also raises an important question to us:

Clinicians must pay attention to and study the prevention and treatment measures of postoperative recurrence and metastasis to improve the efficacy of postoperative remote frame and peroid.

From 1985 to 1999, we conducted a series of animal experimental research and clinical experimental research, review, analysis, and reflection on cancer, summarizing and analyzing the experience and lessons of the pros and cons of success and failure.

So we compiled the above experimental research and clinical practice review, reflection, and analysis of scientific research materials, summarized, compiled, and published the first monograph "New Understanding and New Model of Cancer Therapy", published in January 2001 in China.

2. The second stage
(After 2001)

The research goal and the "target" of cancer treatment are positioned in anti-metastasis, and the key to cancer treatment is anti-metastasis.

After 2001, our research work deeply analyzed what is the key to postoperative recurrence and metastasis?

Looking back to the 1970s, in view of the high rate of recurrence and metastasis after cancer surgery, in order to **prevent recurrence and metastasis after surgery**, a series of postoperative adjuvant chemotherapy was used, and chemotherapy was even started before surgery. But the result is not satisfactory.

Recurrence and metastasis still occur soon after surgery, or metastasis while chemotherapy, the more chemotherapy the more metastasis.

In some cases, intensive chemotherapy has contributed to immune failure. These are all worthy of our clinical teachers to seriously and objectively think and analyze how to prevent recurrence and anti-metastasis in cancer treatment to obtain good long-term treatment effects.

Today, the most important problem in cancer treatment is how to resist metastasis. Metastasis has become a bottleneck in cancer treatment. If the problem of metastasis after radical resection of the patient's cancer cannot be solved, cancer treatment will not be able to leapfrog forward.

Therefore, the key to current cancer research is to resist metastasis. The core topic of cancer treatment is to solve metastasis and recurrence.

One of the keys to cancer treatment is to fight cancer metastasis.

Metastasis is just a phenomenon.

How is it to clearly understand the process, steps and mechanism of cancer cell metastasis?

We should try to understand:

1. *Why do cancer cells metastasize?*
2. *How is it transferred?*
3. *What are the steps, route, process shape, and fate of the transfer?*
4. *What is the molecular mechanism of cancer cell metastasis?*
5. *Where is the weak link in the metastasis of cancer cells?*
6. *Which link or link can be attacked or blocked to achieve the purpose of anti-transfer?*

We have spent more than 3 years experimenting with animal models of cancer metastasis, observing and tracking the regularity of cancer cells in the process of metastasis, looking for ways to disturb and prevent the metastasis of cancer cells.

Through the review, analysis and evaluation of a large number of cases in clinical practice, we proposed:

① *The key to current cancer research is to resist metastasis;*

② *Cancer manifests in three forms in the human body, and the third form is cancer cells on the way of metastasis;*

③ *The goal of cancer treatment should be aimed at these three forms;*

④ *The "two points and one line theory" of the whole process of cancer onset in cancer treatment should not only pay attention to two points, but also pay attention to cutting off the first line;*

⑤ *The specific measures to find anti-metastasis should be to capture, chase, block, and intercept cancer cells during metastasis.*

The third area of anti-cancer metastasis therapy is proposed. The "main battlefield" for annihilating cancer cells during metastasis is in the blood circulation.

It is important to improve immune regulation and control and immunity surveillance, or the important thing is to improve immune regulation and immune surveillance.

By 2005, we compiled a large amount of the above experimental research and clinical verification materials, and summarized, collected and published the monograph "New Concepts and New Methods of Cancer Metastasis Treatment". In April 2007, the book was won the Award of "Three Hundreds" Original Book Title issued by the General Administration of Press and Publishing House of the People's Republic of China.

3. The third stage (After 2006)

It was to focus <u>the main research point</u> on <u>the research of *prevention and treatment* of the whole process of cancer occurrence and development</u>

It was to closely integrate clinical practice, and propose reforms and innovations, scientific research and development in response to the problems and drawbacks of traditional clinical therapies. *It was to recognize that the strategy of cancer prevention and treatment must move forward, the way out for cancer treatment lies in the "three early or three earliest", and the way out for anti-cancer lies in prevention.*

The second monograph is the book that further develops on the basis of the scientific research results from the first monograph, and positions or locates that the "target" of cancer treatment was in anti-metastasis, **which it is very correct to point out that the key to cancer treatment is anti-metastasis.**

However, metastasis is only the last stage of cancer occurrence and development. It is only a local problem during the whole process of cancer occurrence. It cannot reduce the incidence of cancer and may reduce the mortality rate.

After 2006, we realized that it is necessary that the goal of cancer treatment is to focus on the treatment of severely ill patients with the middle and later metastases stages, but the efficacy is very poor. The more new patients, the more patients are treated. Once they are diagnosed, they are in the middle and late stages. The curative effect is not good.

If we want to overcome cancer, it must have "three early" and must be prevented to reduce the incidence of cancer and the death rate of cancer.

<u>The way out for cancer treatment lies in the "three early", and the research on the "three early" must be strengthened.</u>

<u>The occurrence and development of cancer go through the susceptible stage-----precancerous lesions-----invasive stage,</u>

<u>At present, cancer treatments in oncology departments or tumor centers in various cancer hospitals or major hospitals in our country and our province are mainly concentrated in the middle and advanced stages, and the treatment effect is poor. If patients in the middle and late stages can be operated on, they will be treated with surgery. If they cannot, they can only be treated with an appease or conservative or estimated interest rate therapy.</u>

<u>Therefore, the way out for cancer treatment should be in the "three early ", early detection, early diagnosis, and early treatment.</u>

<u>The early-stage patients generally have better treatment effects so that it Improves the treatment effects, which it will inevitably reduce cancer mortality.</u>

<u>Therefore, we must pay attention to the study of early diagnosis methods and treatment methods, and we must also pay attention to the treatment of precancerous lesions, in order to reduce the invasion stage of the middle and advanced patients.</u>

If it can treat the precancerous lesions or early stage cancers well, the number of intermediate and advanced patients who have progressed to invasion and metastasis will be reduced, thus which it will reduce the incidence of cancer.

Therefore, it is believed that the current cancer hospitals or oncology departments in various places mainly treat patients in the middle and advanced stages.

Even if the treatment results are good, they can only reduce the mortality rate, while ignoring the precancerous lesions in the vulnerable or *susceptible stage* or the patients in the early stage, it cannot reduce cancer incidence or occurrence rate, so it is believed *that it must pay attention to the prevention and treatment of the whole process of the occurrence and development of cancer, which is the overall concept of strategic significance.*

We must update our thinking and change our concept.

Dr. Xu Ze has been engaged in oncology surgery for 60 years. It is found that there are more and more patients, and the incidence of cancer is also rising. It is deeply to understand that cancer must not only pay attention to treatment, but also pay attention to prevention, in order to stop at the source.

Therefore, it is to deeply understand that the way out for cancer treatment is in the "three earlys' ", and the research on the "*three earlys'" (early detection, early diagnosis, and early treatment) must be strengthened*.

The way out for anti-cancer lies in prevention, and the study of preventive measures must be strengthened.

As mentioned above, shifting the focus of tumor prevention and treatment strategy forward has two implications as the following:

One is *to change lifestyles*, improve environmental pollution and other preventive measures, <u>and the other is to treat precancerous lesions to prevent their development</u> to the aggressive or middle-to-late stage.

<u>**The way out for cancer control lies in prevention:**</u>

<u>**Research on preventive measures must be strengthened.**</u>

Cancer has become the world's largest public health problem. Compared with other chronic diseases, cancer prevention and control will face greater challenges.

In the past 60 years, cancer deaths in China have shown a significant upward trend, and they have become the number one cause of death among urban and rural residents. On average, 1 in 4 deaths is due to cancer.

Cancer is not only a serious threat to human health, but also an important factor in the monthly increase in medical expenses. The annual direct cost of cancer treatment in my country is nearly 100 billion RMB. It makes patients and the entire society bear a huge economic burden. Many patients have spent tens of thousands or even hundreds of thousands of dollars, but have not achieved the corresponding curative effect. As a result, people and money are exhausted, and cancer mortality is still the first.

What should it be done?

It is worthy of analysis and reflection by our clinicians and should be studied.

How does the research road go?

It must be aware of the current problems in treatment.

Although many countries have invested a lot of money in the treatment of cancer patients, the 5-year survival rate of some common cancers has not improved significantly in the past 30 years.

How should and could it be done?

The way out for cancer control lies in prevention, and the prevention and intervention are the topmost priorities in the public sector.

In recent years, it has been recognized that more than 90% of cancers are caused by environmental factors. *Protecting and restoring a good environment is an important part of cancer prevention. One-third of cancers are preventable.*

The relationship between the environment and cancer is extremely close. Environmental pollution can cause various carcinogens to enter the human body or various carcinogenic factors affect the human body.

How is it to prove the relationship between environmental pollution?

There are many examples in history which has been confirming these relationship.

1. *Air pollution in environmental pollution can be used to increase the incidence of lung cancer*.

Harmful gases such as power generation, steelmaking, automobiles, airplanes, fuels, energy sources, measurement smoke and dust are emitted into the atmosphere in industrialized developed countries, polluting the air, leading to increased incidence and mortality of lung cancer.

2. In environmental pollution, water pollution and cancer, water quality pollution is caused by industrial and agricultural production and urban sewage. Water pollution can induce or promote the occurrence of cancer.

Chemical carcinogenesis in environmental pollution is closely related to the incidence of cancer. 80-90% of human cancers are related to environmental factors, mainly chemical factors.

That studying the sources of environmental pollution carcinogens and studying how to eliminate such pollution is a very important issue for cancer prevention.

The prevention of cancer must prevent pollution.

This thinking and understanding are consistent with today's goals of energy conservation, emission reduction, pollution prevention, and construction of a "**two-oriented society**"(**the environment friendly and the save of resource energy),** and the content is consistent.

Therefore, *it is to consider or think that energy conservation, emission reduction, pollution prevention and treatment are actually the first-level prevention of cancer, which prevents the occurrence of cancer at the source.*

It is to believe that this is a great opportunity to "conquer cancer". It is deeply convinced that building a "two-oriented society" will achieve the role of cancer prevention and cancer control at the same time and obtain good results, so that the people will stay healthy and stay away from cancer.

In order to conquer cancer and conduct cancer prevention and control research, it is necessary to conduct basic and clinical research on anti-cancer metastasis and recurrence, and conduct multidisciplinary collaboration and joint research. It is necessary to establish the Wuhan Anti-Cancer Research Association.

With the strong support of Academician Qiu Fazu, Professor Xu Ze, Li Huiqiao and other professors applied for preparation which was approved by the higher authorities of Taiyi City, the Wuhan Anti-Cancer Research Society was established on June 21, 2009, and then professional committee of the treatment of cancer metastasis and recurrence was established. Then, it was to form cancer metastasis academic research team, academic research, academic seminars, academic publicity, academic workshops or academic seminars, which have cultivated a group of young and middle-aged anti-cancer metastasis and treatment senior talents for our province and our city.

The goals of controlling cancer research:

The foothold is "research".

Under the guidance of the scientific concept of development, with the vision of development, the spirit of innovation, looking forward, facing the future, developing medicine, researching cancer prevention and control, researching the occurrence and development of cancer, cancer metastasis, and searching the mechanism of recurrence and prevention and treatment.

The research route is to discover the problem → ask the question → research the problem → solve the problem or explain the problem in order to help overcome cancer.

In Wuhan, the Wuhan Anti-Cancer Research Association, and the 8+1 hospitals in the Wuhan Metropolitan Area formed the Wuhan Metropolitan Area 8+1 Anti-Cancer Alliance to conduct academic seminars and academic exchanges on cancer prevention and control.

The Wuhan Anti-Cancer Research Society went to Houston, USA to visit the Sterling Oncology Institute for academic exchanges in December 2009, and presented the second monograph "New Concepts and New Methods of Cancer Metastasis Treatment" and "Carcinoma Metastasis Experimental Research Atlas".

By 2010, we have compiled the above experimental and clinical research data, summarized, compiled, and published the third monograph "New Concepts and New Methods of Cancer Treatment" in China version in 2011.

The third monograph (New Concepts and New Methods of Cancer Treatment" is a brand-new concept and innovative content. It has both experimental research basis and clinically verified "New Concepts of Cancer Therapy". It was to propose a series of reforms and innovations in cancer treatment.

With the publication of this new book, happily builds a "two-oriented society", which is conducive to adhere to the innovative path of cancer prevention and control in the "two-oriented society" with Chinese characteristics under the guidance of the scientific development concept.

Since 2013 there are the following continuous publications as:

1. **<<Conquer cancer and launch the total attack to cancer>> in 2018 by Authorhouse In presses in Bloomington, IN in USA**
2. **<<Walked out of the new road to conquer cancer>> Volume II in 2019 by Authorhouse in presses in Bloomington, IN in USA**
3. **<<Walked out of the new road to conquer cancer>> Volume III in 2019 by Authorhouse in presses in Bloomington, IN in USA**
4. **<<The research on anticancer traditional chinese medication with immune regulation and control>> Volume IV in 2019 by Authorhouse in presses in Bloomington, IN in USA**
5. **<<Innovation on clinical application theory of cancer prevention and treatment research in the 21st century>> Volume V in 2019 by Authorhouse in presses in Bloomington, IN in USA**
6. **<< Build up the multidisciplinary and the science city of the research base with related to cancer research for conquering cancer>> Volume VI in 2019 by Authorhouse in presses in Bloomington, IN in USA**
7. **<< Create the researvh institute of the environmental protection>> Volume VII in 2019 by Authorhouse in presses in Bloomington, IN in USA**
8. **<< Create an environmental protection and cancer prevention research institute and carry out cancer prevention system engineering>> Volume VIII in 2019 by Authorhouse in presses in Bloomington, IN in USA**
9. **<<New concepts and new way of treatment of cancer metastasis>> in 2016 by Authorhouse in presses in Bloomington, IN in USA**
10. **<<The new progress in cancer treatment>> in 2018 by Authorhouse in presses in Bloomington, IN in USA**
11. **<<New concept and new way of treatment of cancer>> in 2013 by Authorhouse in presses in Bloomington, IN in USA**

12. <<The road to overcome cancer >> in 2016 by Authorhouse in presses in Bloomington, IN in USA

13. <<On innovation of treatment of cancer>> in 2015 by Authorhouse in presses in Bloomington, IN in USA

14. << Condense Visdom and conquer cancer>> Volume I in 2018 by Authorhouse in presses in Bloomington, IN in USA

15. <<Condense Visdom and conquer cancer>> Volume II in 2018 by Authorhouse in presses in Bloomington, IN in USA

8

Briefly describe the results of anti-cancer research and scientific researches(about Dr. Xu Ze and Dr. Bin Wu)

1. Dr. Xu Ze works hard daily and set up the great models for us to learn from him such as:

He published cancer research monographs, 18 monographs, 15 English edition published in Washington, international distribution

Professor Xu Ze continues to conduct scientific research after his retirement. The scientific journey has not stopped, and the following series of scientific research results have been achieved:

He had an acute myocardial infarction in December 1991. After being rescued and hospitalized for half a year, he gradually recovered. He can no longer undergo surgery. He calmed down and hid in a small building to conduct basic and clinical cancer research.

In 1996, he was 63 years old and retired. After retiring, he has lived in the small building for 20 years. He has been working alone and alone. He continued to conduct a series of experimental studies and clinical verification observations, and achieved the following series of scientific research results.

After more than 20 years of hard work in the cold and heat, a series of experimental research and clinical verification work have been carried out. It is based on my review, analysis, reflection, and experience of clinical cases over the past 60 years, and the results and findings of my own more than 10 years of cancer research. From experiment to clinical, and from clinical to experiment, experimental research and clinical verification data are sorted, summarized, and three monographs have been published.

These 18 monographs are the results of three different scientific research stages and three different levels of our arduous journey, arduous climb, and scientific research step by step.

It was to briefly describe the research results of cancer: the publications and meeting reporting(he also took part in many surgical text book writing).

The publications of monographs on cancer research are as the followings:

1. An Atlas "Experimental study of anticarcinoma recurrence and metastasis"

2. The book

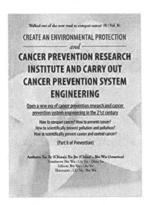

3. **The road to overcome cancer**

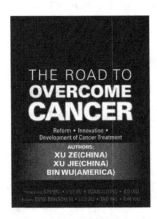

4. Walked out of the new road to conquer cancer

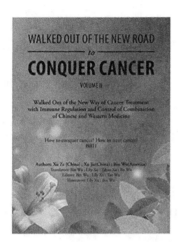

5. New concept and new way of treatment of cancer metastasis

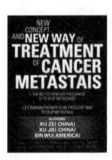

6. On Innovation of treatment of cancer

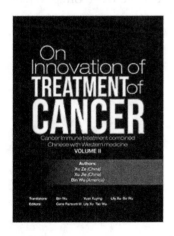

7. Innovation on clinical application theory of cancer prevention

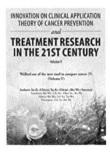

8. Create the research institute of the environmental protection and cancer prevention and carry out cancer prevention system engineering

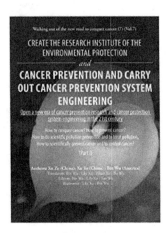

9. Build up the multidisciplinary and the science city of the research base with related to cancer research for conquering cancer

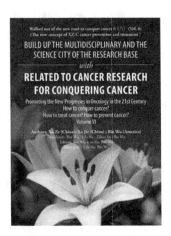

10. New concept and new way of treatment of cancer

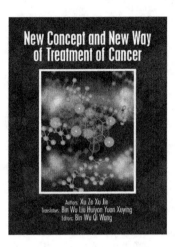

11. The research on anticancer traditional chinese medication with immune regulation and control

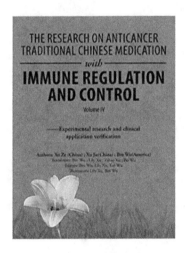

12. alked out of the new road to conquer cancer

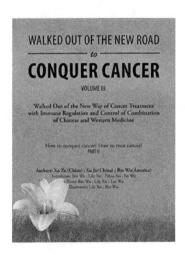

13. The new progress in cancer treatment

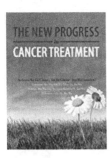

14. Condense wisdom and conquer cancer Part I

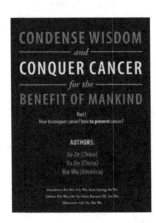

15. Condense wisdom and conquer cancer Part II

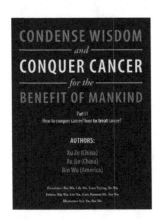

16. Conquer cancer and launch the total attack to cancer

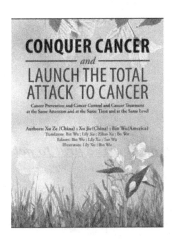

2. Dr. Bin Wu :

She had her M.D and Ph.D degree with the excellent academic score and started her research path since her young age with her father in China. She is very dedicating the human being health study and work. She took part in the book <<Cytomegalovirus(CMV)>> in 2012(she wrote the chapter about immune therapy for CM virus) and she works hard for the human being health day and night.

These 19 monographs are the results of three different scientific research stages and three different levels of our arduous journey, arduous climb, and scientific research step by step.

After all, we are continuing to work hard.

The awards from the following:

Three hundred, original books

Original publishing

The Chinese People's Common and People's Army and Civil Press

The meeting and Poster during the meeting:

Dr. Bin Wu presented several cancer research papers at the American International Oncology Conference [during the AACR (American Association for Cancer Research) meeting], such as: 1. Thymic atrophy and decreased immunologic function:possible factor behind cancer development: 2. Observation of experimental and clinic curative effect on XZ-C medicine treating malignancy, etc totally five papers during AACR meeting.

Immune anti-cancer research

a. The research question:

Is the immune system low first and then cancer easily occures, or is it the first to get cancer and then the immune system decreases later?

b. The experimental results prove:

First, there is a low immunity and then the occurrence and development of cancer. If there is no decline in immune function, it is not easy to succeed in vaccination.

c. The experimental results hint:

Improving and maintaining good immune function is one of the important measures to prevent cancer.

World-class tumor immunologists and clinical oncologists such as Stanford University School of Medicine, University of California at San Francisco, Harvard University School of Medicine, and other world-class tumor immunologists and clinical oncologists fully affirmed Professor Xu Ze's research results, and agreed that

To enhances the anti-replase and anti-metatastasis immunity defense ability of the cancer patients through immune regulation and controlling can fully improve the quality of life of patients with advanced cancer;

It is the most effective anti-cancer approach after surgery therapy, radiotherapy and chemotherapy.

9

Accessories

A. The Letter from Academician

<u>The encouragement and guidance for research directions and research approaches Evaluation and recognition of academic value and academic level are as the following:</u>

Instruction or Pointing out: Letter 1

Traditional Chinese medicine and biological therapy are the two most promising ways to resist metastasis, especially Chinese medicine and traditional Chinese medicine, I hope you will walk out of our country's characteristic Hangzhou transfer road.

Instruction or Pointing out: Letter 2

The model from clinical to experimental, and from experimental to clinical is very good, and it is also very correct to take the road of integrating Chinese and Western medicine.

I sincerely hope that you will keep moving forward and find a new way to overcome cancer.

Hope: Letter 3

I very much agree with your ideas and thoughts on conquering cancer in the book. In particular, you have made a lot of contributions to cancer treatment and clinical research, and I am deeply impressed.

I hope that you can make a breakthrough in Chinese medicine and traditional Chinese medicine, so that the majority of patients can benefit, so that Chinese medicine can be further developed, so that my country's medical industry can step into the world's leading position

Encouragement: Letter 4

Tumors are hard bones to gnaw, but we should continue to do it... As long as it is effective, it will be supported whether it is directly on the tumor, on the body, or reducing the response to radiotherapy and chemotherapy.

Development: Letter 5

The experimental surgery is extremely important in the development of medical science. Our hospital also intends to strengthen the research of experimental surgery, especially the research on tumor treatment.

At that time, we will send people to your institute to study, and welcome to give lectures in our institute

B. The evaluation and demonstration of academic value and academic level: (the abbreviations of the original)

1. FACULTY OF MEDICINE

From CHINESE UNIVERSITY OF HONG KONG

XXX had read the book you sent [New Concept and New Method of Cancer Metastasis Treatment]. I very much agree with the concepts and thinking that you put forward in the book to overcome cancer. In particular, you have made a lot of contributions to the basic and clinical research of cancer treatment and I am deeply impressed.

There are many domestic researches on the treatment of cancer with Chinese medicine, especially the combination of Chinese and Western medicine, but the data you have obtained through a large number of animal experiments are rare. Traditional Chinese medicine is a huge treasure left by our ancestors. Only through the efforts of our generation can further development be achieved. I hope you can make more efforts in this area to bring Chinese medicine treatment to a new peak.

Evidence-based medicine is the general trend and accepted direction of the international medical community. The future development of traditional Chinese medicine must be accepted by a wide range of people only through scientific and systematic research.

I understand that the basic medical theories of Chinese medicine and Western medicine are different, and it is very difficult to apply evidence-based medicine to Chinese medicine. However, if scientific clinical research is not adopted, such as randomized double-blind clinical research, the actual effect of Chinese medicine and traditional Chinese medicine treatment is still doubtful in many people's minds.

I hope you can make breakthrough contributions to Chinese medicine and traditional Chinese medicine, so that the majority of patients can benefit, so that Chinese medicine and traditional Chinese medicine can be further developed, so that my country's medical industry can step into the world's leading position.

Best wishes

xxxxx

Department of Surgery, Chinese University of Hong Kong March 22, 2006

XXX, Professor, Department of Surgery, Chinese University of Hong Kong

2. Zhongshan Hospital Affiliated to Fudan University

Address: Shanghai Fenglinqiao Medical College Road 136
Phone: xxxx
Academician XXXX: Academician of Chinese Academy of Engineering
Academician of the Chinese Academy of Engineering, internationally renowned liver cancer scholar, professor of surgery, doctoral supervisor, Fudan University Affiliated Middle School: Director of the Institute of Liver Cancer, Shan Hospital

National Key Discipline Leader of Oncology, Director of International Union Against Cancer (UICC) and Chairman of Liver Cancer Examination Committee of Chinese Anti-You Association.

3. The state Key Laboratory of Molecular Oncology

XXX: Academician of the Chinese Academy of Sciences, Doctor of Medicine, Professor, Deputy Director of the Department of Biology of the Chinese Academy of Sciences, Director of the Cell Biology Department of the Chinese Academy of

Medical Sciences, and the Cancer Institute of Peking Union Medical College, and Director of the National Key Laboratory of Molecular Oncology.

4. <u>XXXXX, Academician of Chinese Academy of Sciences, Doctor of Medicine: I had been reading your books carefully, which are the high qualities on the new concepts, etc.</u>

Printed in the United States
by Baker & Taylor Publisher Services